Contents

Foreword

As fitness and sport enthusiasts are becoming increasingly educated about exercise in general a demand has emerged for coaches to be more conversant with safe exercise techniques. The modern exercise coach has a moral and professional responsibility to educate and encourage participants to exercise safely and effectively, using their professional knowledge to instil an understanding of what is and what is not correct technique. The author, in writing this book, brings a wealth of expertise and experience drawn personally from many areas of exercise and sport.

This book has been written specifically for any practitioner, professional or coach who is responsible for the teaching of safe and good practice in exercise. The text draws in particular from recent advances in the classical disciplines of strength and toning exercises and effective stretching. In this regard it is important for all coaches to remember that our understanding of this field continues to evolve, and that it is therefore necessary for all fitness professionals and coaches to continue their education and remain updated on all aspects of industry trends and research.

In meeting the continuing thirst for further education in this field *Safe and Effective Exercise* will help to develop an understanding of the factors which constitute a correct exercise technique, as well as to guide those coaches who want to bring out the best in their charges – safely and effectively.

Gillian Cummings-Bell BA (Hons) M.Sc.

Safe and Effective Exercise

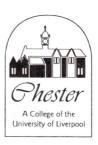
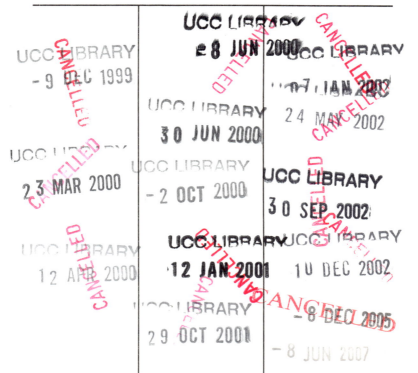

First published in 1998
The Crowood Press Ltd
Ramsbury, Marlborough
Wiltshire SN8 2HR

British Library Cataloguing-in-Publication Data

A catalogue record for this book is available from the British Library.

ISBN 1 86126 169 1

Dedication
To Chris, my wife.

Acknowledgements

I would like to thank the following people for their contributions towards the completion of this book: Gillian Cummings-Bell for her advice and for writing the Foreword; Cherry Baker (Exercise Association Instructor of the Year, 1993–94) for her valuable suggestions and for being an ideal model; Robert Durn for taking the photographs despite a heavy work schedule; Don Scaife (Stockport College Media Services) who also fitted time into a very heavy work schedule to produce the computerised illustrations for Chapter 5; Adidas UK who provided clothing for the photographs.

Typeset by Phoenix Typesetting, Ilkley, West Yorkshire
Printed and bound in Great Britain by WBC Book Manufacturers Ltd., Mid Glamorgan.

Introduction

Why another book on exercise? Well, this is not *just* 'another book' but one with a particular theme: *Safety* and *Effectiveness*.

I see so many people exercising using outdated methods which have since been shown to be potentially dangerous and ineffective. Not only do I see performers themselves executing such moves, but also coaches putting their charges through a battery of controversial and contra-indicated exercises. Some coaches are highly qualified in their own particular sport, but may lack up-to-date knowledge of safe exercise practice, a detailed knowledge of the structure and function of the human body, and how the structure and function of the body is affected by certain exercises. This knowledge is of vital importance for anyone in a position of responsibility for another person's health and physical conditioning.

I am sure that nobody would entrust their car to an unqualified 'mechanic' who lacked essential knowledge. Why then should a person entrust his or her body and health to a person unqualified in that respect?!

It is the duty of any fitness professional to remain up-to-date with current research into the effects of exercise and training. As medical and technical developments progress, individual coaches are expected to keep abreast of relevant changes and modify their coaching practices accordingly. For example, certain warm-up exercises routinely followed by coaches a number of years ago have now been identified as potentially damaging to an athlete's spine. Such discredited exercises should no longer be adopted by coaches since, by doing so they are making themselves vulnerable to an allegation of negligence (Bailey, 1996).

The contents of this book are the result of a lifetime spent in Physical Education and Exercise Sciences. The information enclosed within should be essential knowledge contributing to the qualifications of any exercise teacher, personal trainer, coach, physical education teacher or sports therapist. It should also help those involved in their own exercise training regime, whether they be members of the public involved in a health-related fitness programme, or the serious athlete/sports person involved in rigorous training.

Many people, out of ignorance of correct procedure and knowledge of the body, are exercising inappropriately and incorrectly, causing more harm than good. A statistical study by financial scientists at Sheffield University concluded that the majority of younger people (<40) exercising on a regular basis actually cost the health services more in injury treatment than is saved because of increases in health-related fitness. And this is not to mention the cost to industry and commerce due to time off work. This is fuel for the fires of the anti-exercise brigade, and bad news for those of us trying to promote an active lifestyle. Unfortunately, I have to admit I see no reason to doubt the claims of the Sheffield study, as many of those injuries will occur because of inappropriate and improperly practised exercise. The unfortunate paradox is that many people are exercising for potential health benefits, yet are suffering avoidable conditions because of incorrect exercise practice.

Appropriate and correctly practised exercise should be safe and beneficial. The purpose of this book is to contribute towards a knowledge and awareness of safe and effective exercise, to discuss different methods of exercising and the many different exercises which exist, to point out the dangers, and to illustrate safe and effective practice. It is hoped that the following chapters will provide essential knowledge for exercise participants, trainers, coaches, teachers and sports therapists to enable safe and effective exercises to be performed and enjoyed.

Part One: General Principles

1 The Training Principles

If we look up the word 'principle' in the *Oxford English Dictionary* we find definitions such as a 'truth', a 'general law', a 'law of nature'. We should normally be very reserved about making 'laws' about the body. It is such a complex organism that we cannot always state exactly how it will perform, react, respond and so on. However, when it comes to developing, maintaining or increasing fitness, certain principles apply and cannot be disputed; they are referred to as the 'Training Principles'. They make absolute sense, should be known by anyone involved in the performance of exercise and the development of fitness, and should be observed.

1. *The Principle of Overload* states that if we want to improve the systems of the body (become fitter), we have to subject the body to greater stresses than those to which the body is accustomed.

There can be no argument. If we want to become fitter, we have to exercise. Exercise places stresses on the systems of the body and if the body is not exercised it will not become fitter. If the couch potato does not exercise, he/she will remain a couch potato.

2. *The Principle of Adaptation* states that over a period of time the systems of the body that are regularly stressed will adapt (physiological changes occur in the tissues) and we can then cope with the increased level of stress which becomes normal (we become fitter).

NB: An important aspect of any physical training programme however should be adequate rest and recovery. During actual training *catabolism* takes place (we are actually damaging and breaking down tissue). It is during the rest periods between training sessions that *anabolism* (repair and strengthening) takes place, and therefore recovery periods must be regular and long enough. The body always over-compensates (known as super-compensation). It not only heals and repairs tissue, but repairs it stronger than it was before.

3. *The Principle of Progression* states that if we want to improve the systems of the body even further (become fitter still) we must further overload those systems (train harder – which might involve a higher intensity, a longer duration, a higher frequency or all three).

N.B. We reach a level of fitness through a certain level of training and if the training remains the same we plateau out at that level. If we want to become fitter still we have to increase the training. However, adaptation and increases in fitness only occur if progression is at an achievable rate. Compare progression to climbing stairs or a ladder. Go one step at a time; attempting too many steps too soon could result in injury and break-down. Do not progress too rapidly.

4. *The Principle of Specificity* states that the systems of the body adapt in a specific way according to the particular type of stress imposed.

Simply put, this means that physiological changes (improvements) take place in the specific tissues trained and according to how they are trained; the body becomes specifically fit for the type of activity and the intensity of training regularly carried out.

5. *The Principle of Reversibility* states that if training stops for a period of time (longer than recovery rest for adaptation), the body will revert towards its pre-trained state.

In other words, if we neglect our training for long enough, we will lose our fitness, and if we neglect our specific training we will lose our specific fitness.

2 Anatomy, Physiology and Kinesiology Applied to Exercise

Anatomy is concerned with the *structure* of the body: what it consists of, and identifying and naming the body parts. *Physiology* is concerned with the *function* of the body: how those parts work. Kinesiology involves identifying how the body moves: which joints are moving, which muscles are causing that movement, which joints are static and which muscles stabilize them, which muscles are shortening and which are lengthening — a knowledge essential to anyone involved with the performance, supervision or prescription of exercise.

ANATOMICAL TERMINOLOGY

A number of words are used in anatomy and should be within the vocabulary of exercise professionals:

Anterior – front.
Posterior – back.
Superior – above or higher.
Inferior – below or lower.
Medial – nearer to the mid-line, or inner.
Lateral – away from the mid-line, or outer/to the side.
Proximal – nearer to the main part of the body (e.g. the end of a limb, bone or muscle).
Distal – further from the main part of the body (e.g. the other end of a limb, bone, muscle).
Articulation – joint.
Supine – face up.
Prone – face down.

BONE AND THE SKELETON

For many people, their impression of bone is that of a hard, dead substance found in the butcher's shop, or seen in pictures of deserts and droughts where bleached white bones remain long after the death of an animal. In fact, bone in the human body is living tissue made up of constantly changing cells. It has a blood supply and a nerve supply, requires nutrition and fulfils many functions in the body.

The skeleton provides a *framework* for the body, much like scaffolding or the steel framework of a building; bones provide *attachment points* for muscles which in turn move those bones; bones act as *lever arms* for movement and the application of force; the skeleton also *allows movement* through the existence of joints between the bones; bones are the 'factories' where *blood cells* are produced, and act as a *reservoir for minerals,* especially calcium and phosphorus. Certain bones provide *protection* for vital organs.

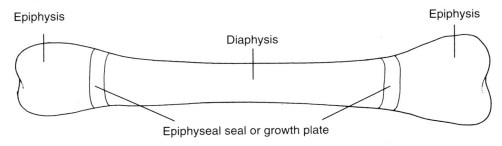

Fig. 1. A typical long bone showing the ossified diaphysis, epiphyses and the growth plates.

Bones are formed before birth but in the form of cartilage. Progressively, during foetal development, and especially during childhood growth, the cartilage cells (chondrocytes) are replaced by bone cells (osteocytes). Eventually, by about the age of 21, all the bones of the body have fully hardened and skeletal maturity is achieved. This hardening of bone is known as *ossification,* although it is sometimes referred to as *calcification.*

The first part of the bone to harden is the central shaft or *diaphysis.* Next the two ends, or *epiphyses,* harden. For a while there remains a comparatively soft section between the hardened epiphyses and the diaphysis known as the *epiphyseal seal,* or *growth plate.* This growth plate consists of mainly cartilage cells and is responsible for an increase in length of the bone during growth spurts (hardened, or ossified, bone

cannot grow; only the softer parts can continue to grow).

Such 'soft' areas in immature bone create potential dangers for youngsters involved in exercise and training. Excesses of repetitive training, or repeated periods of high intensity and high resistance, can distort these growth plates, creating pain and discomfort, especially during the teenage years and even into young adulthood.

Mature bone consists of two parts: the hard, outer layer known as *compact bone,* and a softer inner known as *cancellous tissue,* or *spongy bone.* The latticework construction of bone gives it very high tensile strength and resiliance to withstand great stresses. In fact, like other tissue in the body, bone depends on regular physical stress to maintain its strength and density. Regular exercise therefore is very beneficial to the bones of the

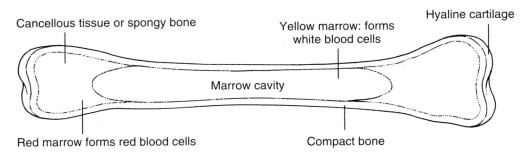

Fig. 2. A section through a typical long bone showing its construction.

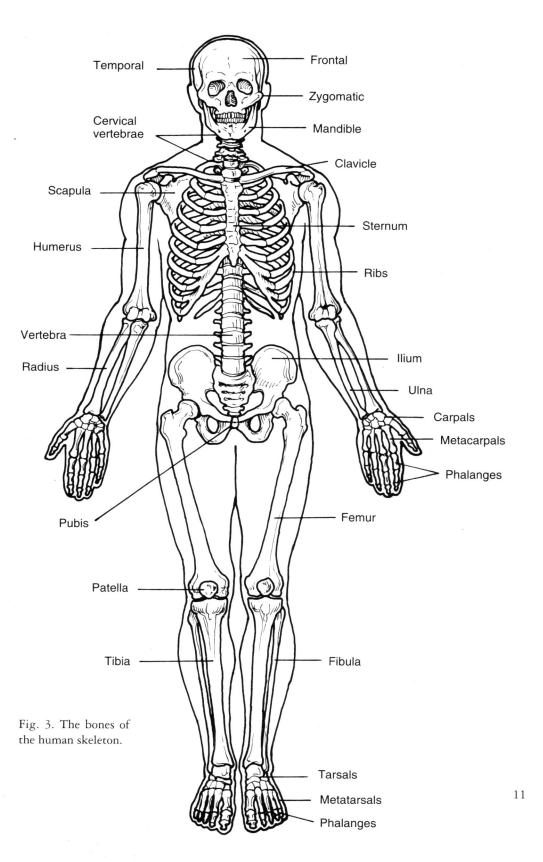

Temporal

Frontal

Zygomatic

Cervical
vertebrae

Mandible

Clavicle

Scapula

Sternum

Humerus

Ribs

Vertebra

Ilium

Radius

Ulna

Carpals

Metacarpals

Phalanges

Pubis

Femur

Patella

Tibia

Fibula

Tarsals

Metatarsals

Phalanges

Fig. 3. The bones of
the human skeleton.

11

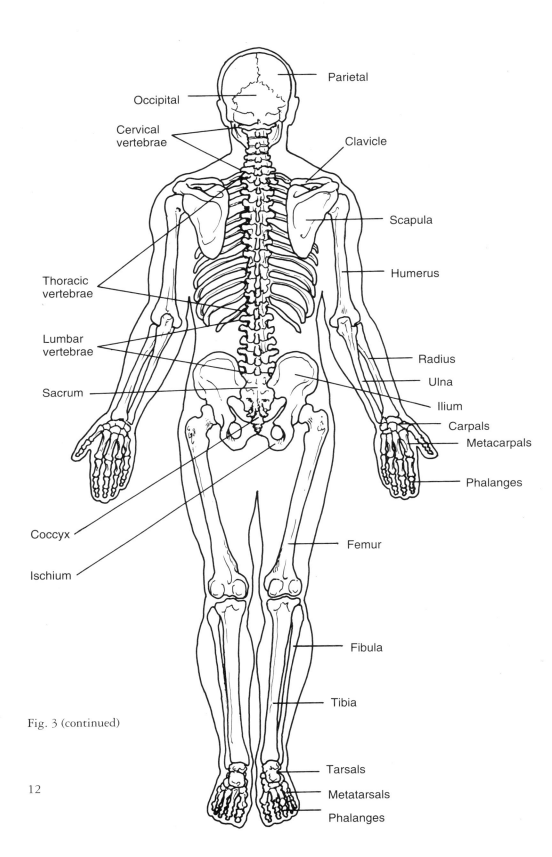

Occipital

Parietal

Cervical
vertebrae

Clavicle

Scapula

Humerus

Thoracic
vertebrae

Lumbar
vertebrae

Radius

Ulna

Sacrum

Ilium

Carpals

Metacarpals

Phalanges

Coccyx

Femur

Ischium

Fibula

Tibia

Tarsals

Metatarsals

Phalanges

Fig. 3 (continued)

12

skeleton as it provides that necessary stress. Of particular benefit is weight-bearing exercise (body weight or additional weight) where muscles exert forces against bones to overcome gravity.

JOINTS

An important aspect of the skeletal system with reference to exercise involves a knowledge of the joints. There are basically two types of joints in the body: *movable* joints and *immovable* joints.

Immovable Joints

Immovable joints employ a pad of fibrous connective tissue between the two bones. Examples can be found in the sutures of the skull. Other immovable joints exist between the upper (proximal) ends of the tibia and fibula of the lower leg, and the sacro-iliac joint at the base of the spine where it articulates with the pelvis. Such joints are not supposed to move, although excesses of stress from very high forces in sport, or repetitive incorrect exercise, can stress those joints and result in inflammation and pain.

Movable Joints

Movable joints can be sub-divided into two types: *slightly movable joints* and *freely movable joints* (*synovial joints*).

Slightly movable joints employ cartilage between the two bones and only slight movement is permitted. Examples of slightly movable joints include the joints between the ribs and sternum, and between the ribs and vertebrae. These joints allow enough movement for the expansion of the thorax during breathing yet still hold a comparatively rigid structure for the protection of vital organs.

Freely movable, or *synovial joints* have a very strong joint capsule composed of tough connective tissue. Within the joint capsule is a synovial membrane which secretes synovial fluid into the joint to lubricate and nourish the joint surface. Strong ligaments connect bone to bone at the joints. They help stabilise the joint and determine the extent of movement range.

Synovial joints can be further classified according to their plane and range of movement, both of which are determined by the shape of the articulating bony surfaces and the ligaments. The different synovial joints include ball and socket, hinge, gliding (or sliding), pivot, condyloid and saddle. Joint movements are

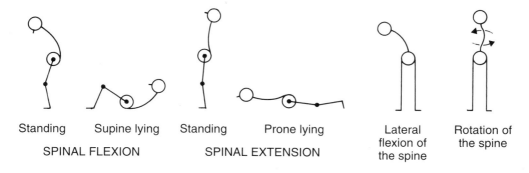

Standing   Supine lying   Standing   Prone lying   Lateral flexion of the spine   Rotation of the spine

SPINAL FLEXION   SPINAL EXTENSION

Fig. 4. Spinal flexion, extension and rotation.

13

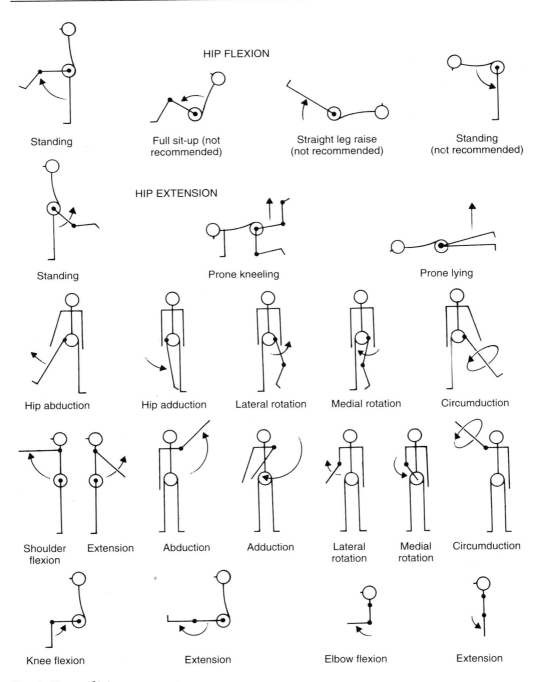

Fig. 5. Types of joint movements.

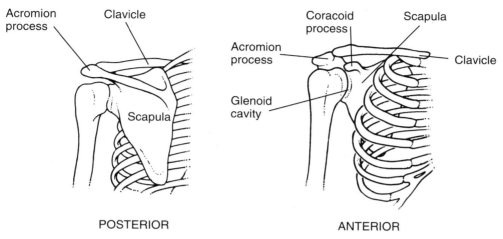

POSTERIOR   ANTERIOR

Fig. 6. The shoulder joint

given particular names: flexion, extension, abduction, adduction, rotation, circumduction.

With reference to exercise, some synovial joints require special consideration.

Ball and socket joints (shoulder, hip) have a great range of movement, although the range of movement at the shoulder is greater than that of the hip because of the presence of the shoulder girdle, the movement of the scapula, and the shallow socket where the head of the humerus articulates with the scapula.

The hip joint has a deep socket and is comparatively stable, whereas the shoulder joint has a very shallow socket and stability is dependent on strong ligaments and strong musculature. Consequently, the shoulder can be easily strained through inappropriate exercise, or dislocated through violent forces.

Ball and socket joints permit all types of joint movement: flexion, extension, abduction, adduction, rotation (medial and lateral) and circumduction.

Hinge joints are capable of movement in one plane only and permit only flexion and extension. Examples include the elbow, the joints

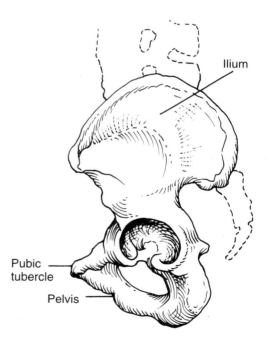

Fig. 7. The hip joint.

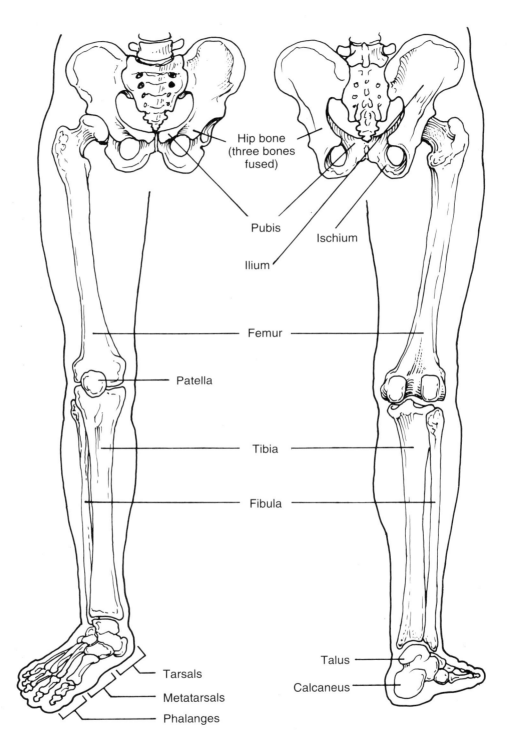

Hip bone
(three bones
fused)

Pubis

Ischium

Ilium

Femur

Patella

Tibia

Fibula

Talus

Calcaneus

Tarsals

Metatarsals

Phalanges

Fig. 7. The hip joint. (continued)

between individual phalanges in the fingers and toes, and, to a lesser extent, the knee joint (between the tibia and femur).

The knee is not a true hinge joint because, although it appears mainly to flex and extend, it is in fact capable of some rotation. When the knee is locked out (hyperextension) slight rotation occurs between the tibia and the femur. This has implications for safety with certain exercises and standing positions. With repetitive movements or standing positions, which involve high compressive forces through the knee joint, locking out should be avoided because of the shearing force which occurs in the semi-lunar cartilages (menisci) between the joint surfaces. Also, repetitive hyperflexion of this joint can result in the joint being progressively forced open and excessive strain imposed on the ligaments which attempt to stabilize the joint.

Gliding or *sliding joints* involve two flat, bony surfaces which slide over each other. An example of these are the facet joints between adjacent vertebrae of the spine. Repeated ballistic hyperextension of the spine can cause friction and wear on the articulating surface, resulting in inflammation of these joints.

Pivot joints allow rotation to occur. Examples include the joint between the top two cervical (neck) vertebrae (atlas and axis), the proximal joint between the radius and ulna near the elbow which allows supination and pronation of the hand (these movements do not come from the wrist which is a condyloid joint), and between the bodies of certain adjacent vertebrae. Ballistic rotations of the trunk create a momentum which takes the vertebral joints to their limit, tugging at the tiny ligaments which can cause trauma and inflammation.

It should be obvious that there are a number

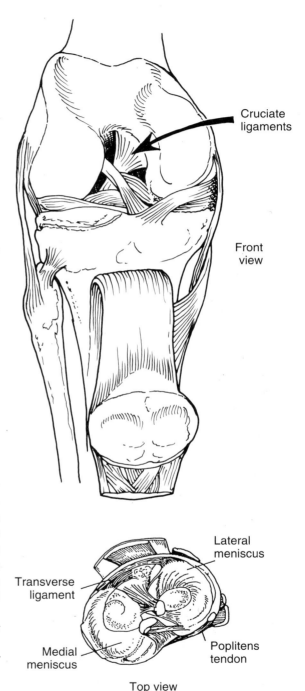

Cruciate ligaments

Front view

Lateral meniscus

Transverse ligament

Medial meniscus

Poplitens tendon

Top view

Fig. 8. The knee joint.

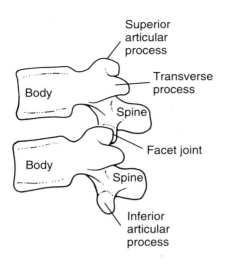
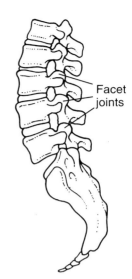

Fig. 9. Facet joints of the spine.

of different types of joint present in the vertebral column. Despite great strength and resilience, the spinal joints can be subjected to excessive stresses by repetitive and ballistic forward and lateral flexion and, as mentioned, by repetitive and ballistic hyperextension or rotation.

MUSCLES

Skeletal muscle is contractile: that is, a muscle causes movement by contraction (shortening) and pulling the bone to which it is attached. Although muscles lengthen they do not push. By lengthening they control movement. Muscles are attached to bones by tendons. The attachment points of muscles are referred to as the *origin* and the *insertion*. The origin is the more fixed end, and the insertion is the end attached to the bone which moves.

A muscle is wrapped in a sheath of connective tissue known as *epimysium*. The muscle is made

up of bundles of fibres wrapped in connective tissue known as *perimysium*. Each fibre is made up of bundles of *myofybrils* wrapped in connective tissue. Each myofybril is made up of *protein filaments* of *actin* and *myosin*. A group of filaments is known as a *sarcomere*. Skeletal muscle is also known as *striped* muscle because its make-up gives it a striped appearance under the microscope. It is also *voluntary* muscle because it is under our conscious control.

It is the *sliding action* of the actin and myosin filaments which causes the muscle as a whole to contract and to develop tension. This tension can then generate force to overcome resistances or create movement.

The amount of tension developed in a muscle is determined by the number of fibres contracting. Skeletal muscles are stimulated by impulses from *motor nerves* which contain many *motor neurones* (nerve cells). Each motor neurone stimulates a number of muscle fibres, either just a few or a few thousand. The motor neurone and the fibres it stimulates are known as a *motor unit*.

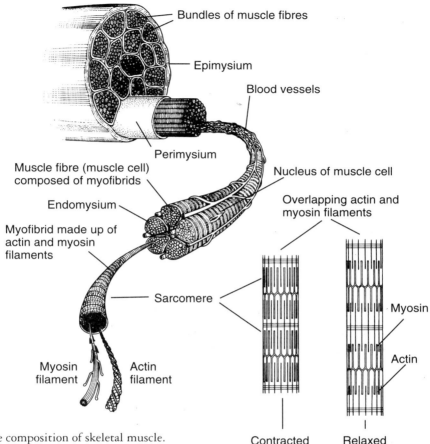

Fig. 10. The composition of skeletal muscle.

Muscles work in pairs known as *opposing muscles* or *antagonistic pairs*. The movement of any joint requires at least two muscles to work at the same time, one shortening and the other lengthening. This phenomenon whereby the nervous system stimulates two muscles simultaneously but to work in opposite directions is known as *reciprocal innervation*.

The muscle shortening to cause the movement is known as the *prime mover*. The muscle lengthening to control the movement is the *antagonist*.

When a muscle *shortens* to cause movement it is involved in *concentric contraction*. When a muscle *lengthens* to control a movement it is involved in *eccentric contraction*. Eccentric contraction may sometimes be referred to as *relaxation*. True relaxation of a muscle involves the muscle lengthening with minimum tension developing. Eccentric contraction usually involves some degree of tension as the fibres attempt to hold back against a (usually lowering/with gravity) force.

Both concentric and eccentric contractions are

19

isotonic contractions because muscle tension results in movement of a joint. If there is muscle tension and there is no movement of a joint (static), it is known as *isometric contraction*.

Most recommended health-related strengthening and toning exercises involve isotonic contractions. The muscle being worked during the 'effort' or 'positive' phase is working as a prime mover and is involved in concentric contraction. During the return phase it is involved in eccentric contraction.

The biceps muscle acting as a prime mover is involved in concentric contraction during elbow flexion, and eccentric contraction during elbow extension (when the forearm is lowered [e.g. return of a 'curl']).

As well as acting as prime movers or antagonists, muscles can also act as *synergists* and *fixators*. Synergists are muscles which *help or assist*. A *true synergist* will assist the prime mover to cause the movement (for example, brachioradialis [front of forearm, crossing the elbow] assists the prime movers biceps and brachialis during elbow flexion).

A muscle may also assist a prime mover by fixing a joint that one end of the prime mover crosses and which would therefore be moved by the prime mover. For example, certain muscles will fix the shoulder joint so that the biceps can flex the elbow. The biceps also crosses the shoulder joint and so that joint must be fixed so that the biceps does not move it. The muscles which fix the shoulder so that the biceps can flex the elbow are known as fixator synergists.

True fixators fix (stabilize) joints in other parts of the body not necessarily affected by the prime mover. For example, during a press-up the joints moving are the shoulders and elbows. The pectorals and the triceps are the prime mover muscles. However, other muscles must fix and hold steady the hips, knees, ankles and spinal joints.

Muscles have a *range*, from fully lengthened to fully contracted (full range). As muscles move joints, the joints are therefore moved through the same range. If a muscle contracts through its full range, then the joint will move through its full range. Muscles and joints can also move through sections of their full range.

For health-related fitness, with the exception of the abdominals, it is generally recommended that all muscles and joints are worked through their full range and not repetitively through a part of that range.

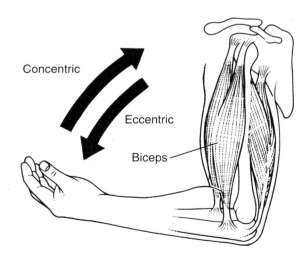

Concentric

Eccentric

Biceps

Fig. 11. The biceps muscle.

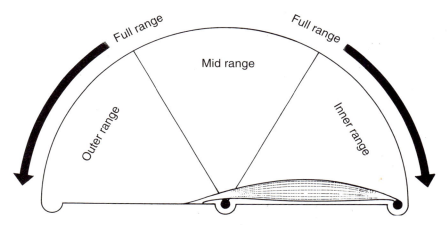

Fig. 12. Muscle and joint range (e.g. a typical hinge joint such as the elbow flexed by Biceps).

A knowledge of the major muscles of the body is essential, along with a knowledge of the joints they cross, their attachment points, and the movements they cause:

Upper Body Muscles

BICEPS (front of the upper arm)
Origin – Above the shoulder joint.
Insertion – Tuberosity of radius (crosses both the elbow and shoulder joints).
Action – Flexion of the elbow, supination of the forearm, flexion of the shoulder as a synergist if the shoulder is not fixed.

BRACHIALIS (front of the upper arm, under the biceps)
Origin – Half-way down the anterior humerus.
Insertion – Proximal end of the ulna (crosses only the elbow joint).
Action – Flexion of the elbow.

TRICEPS (back of the upper arm)
Origin – Three heads: Long head – above the shoulder joint on the scapula; Lateral head –

proximal posterior surface of humerus; Short head – lower posterior surface of humerus.
Insertion – Proximal end of the ulna.
Action – Extension of the elbow, extension of the shoulder as a synergist if the shoulder is not fixed.

PECTORALIS MAJOR (chest)
Origin – Sternum.
Insertion – By wide tendon to the upper anterior surface of the humerus.
Action – Most movements of the shoulder, especially horizontal adduction, flexion, vertical adduction, medial rotation of the humerus.

TRAPEZIUS (neck, shoulders and upper back)
Origin – Base of skull, seventh cervical vertebrae, thoracic vertebrae.
Insertion – Posterior clavicle, spine of scapula.
Action – Elevation of the scapula (shrugging the shoulder), adduction of the scapula, fixation of the scapula.

RHOMBOIDS (upper back between the thoracic spine and the scapulae)

21

Origin – Last cervical and first five thoracic vertebrae.

Insertion – Medial border of the scapula.

Action – Pulls the scapula towards the spine, downwards rotation of the scapula.

DELTOID (top of the shoulder)

Origin – Outer part of the clavicle, spine of the scapula.

Insertion – Upper lateral surface of the humerus.

Action – Abduction of the shoulder joint (lifts the arm up), also some flexion and horizontal adduction of the shoulder (anterior fibres), horizontal abduction of the shoulder (posterior fibres).

LATISSIMUS DORSI (back)

Origin – Top of the posterior ilium, back of the sacrum, lumbar and lower six thoracic vertebrae, and lower three ribs.

Insertion – Medial side of upper end of the humerus.

Action – Shoulder adduction, horizontal abduction, extension and medial rotation.

ERECTOR SPINAE (back)

Origin – Posterior crest of the ilium, sacrum, lower seven ribs, lumbar vertebrae, thoracic vertebrae.

Insertion – Ribs, all vertebrae, base of the skull.

Action – Extension of the spine, lateral flexion of the spine (one side, together with abdominals and quadratus lumborum).

Abdominals

RECTUS ABDOMINIS

Origin – Crest of pubis.

Insertion – Costal cartilage of fifth, sixth and seventh ribs, lower end of the sternum (xiphoid process).

Action – Trunk flexion and lateral flexion.

INTERNAL OBLIQUES

Origin – Inguinal ligament, anterior iliac crest,
lumbar fascia.

Insertion – eighth, ninth and tenth ribs, linea alba.

Action – Rotates and flexes the trunk (right side of muscle to the right, left side of muscle to the left).

EXTERNAL OBLIQUES

Origin – Lower eight ribs.

Insertion – Anterior iliac crest, inguinal ligament, pubis, fascia of rectus abdominis.

Action – Rotates and flexes the trunk (right side of muscle to the left, left side of muscle to the right).

TRANSVERSE ABDOMINIS

Origin – Inguinal ligament, anterior iliac crest, lower six ribs, lumbar fascia.

Insertion – Crest of the pubis, linea alba.

Action – Abdominal posture, forced expiration (transverse abdominis does not cross or move a joint. It is worked by exhaling and by pulling in the abdomen).

Hip Flexors (lumbar, groin and pelvic region)

ILIACUS

Origin – Inner surface of the ilium.

Insertion – Lesser trochanter of the femur.

Action – Flexion of the hip.

PSOAS MAJOR

Origin – Twelfth thoracic vertebra and all lumbar vertebrae.

Insertion – Lesser trochanter of the femur.

Action – Flexion of the hip.

NB Iliacus and psoas major share the same attachment point (insertion) on the femur and work together to cause hip flexion. They are often referred to collectively as iliopsoas.

Hip Extensors

GLUTEUS MAXIMUS (buttock)
Origin – Posterior iliac crest, sacrum and lumbar fascia.
Insertion – Upper end of the femur and iliotibial band.
Action – Extension of the hip.

Quadriceps Group (front of thigh)

VASTUS LATERALIS
Origin – Lateral aspect of the femur below greater trochanter and lateral shaft of the femur.
Insertion – By the quadriceps/patella tendon to the tibial tuberosity.
Action – Extension of the knee.

VASTUS INTERMEDIUS
Origin – Upper anterior femur.
Insertion – By the quadriceps/patella tendon to the tibial tuberosity.
Action – Extension of the knee.

VASTUS MEDIALIS
Origin – Medial shaft of the femur.
Insertion – By the quadriceps/patella tendon to the tibial tuberosity.
Action – Extension of the knee.

RECTUS FEMORIS
Origin – Anterior-inferior iliac spine.
Insertion – By the quadriceps/patella tendon to the tibial tuberosity.
Action – Extension of the knee, flexion of the hip.

Hamstrings (back of thigh)

SEMITENDINOSUS (medial)
Origin – Tuberosity of the ischium.
Insertion – Upper anterior medial condyle of the tibia.
Action – Flexion of the knee, extension of the hip, medial rotation of the hip and knee.

SEMIMEMBRANOSUS (medial)
Origin – Tuberosity of the ischium.
Insertion – Posterior medial condyle of the tibia.
Action – Flexion of the knee, extension of the hip, medial rotation of the hip and knee.

BICEPS FEMORIS (lateral)
Origin – Two heads; tuberosity of the ischium, posterior shaft of the femur.
Insertion – Lateral condyle of the tibia and head of the fibula.
Action – Flexion of the knee, extension of the hip, lateral rotation of the hip and knee.

Adductor Muscles (inner thigh)

ADUCTOR BREVIS, ADDUCTOR LONGUS, ADDUCTOR MAGNUS, GRACILIS
Origin – Pubis and ischium tuberosity.
Insertion – Various sites along the shaft of the the femur. (Gracilis attaches to the anterior medial head of the tibia.)
Action – Adduction of the hip; brevis and magnus also laterally rotate the hip; longus assists with flexion of the hip; gracilis assists with flexion of the knee and medial rotation of the hip.

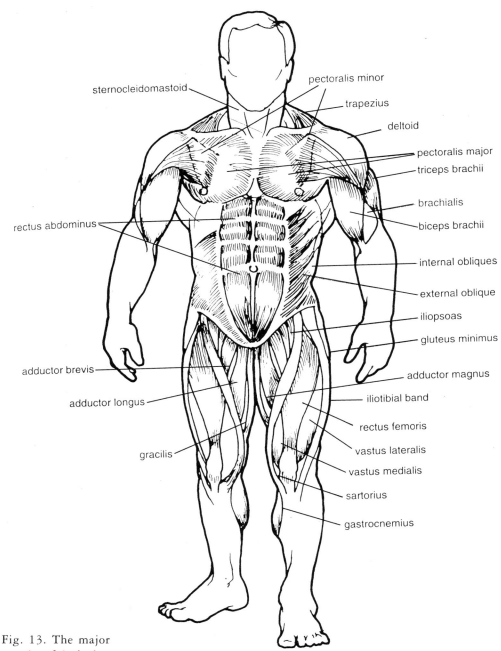

Fig. 13. The major
muscles of the body.

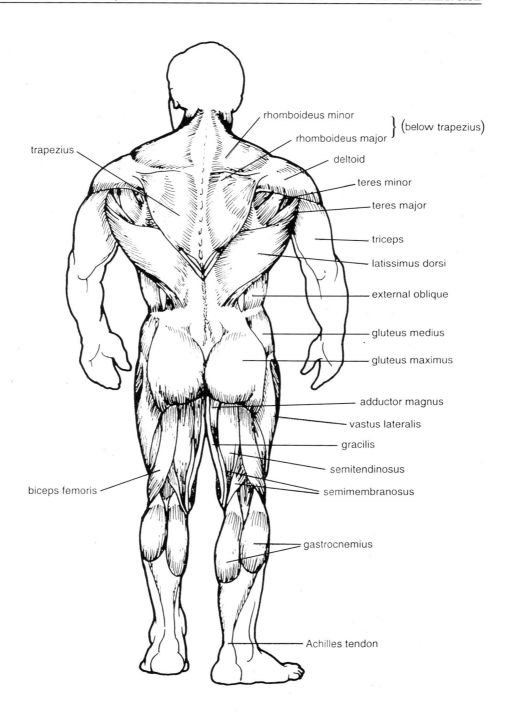

rhomboideus minor
rhomboideus major } (below trapezius)
trapezius
deltoid
teres minor
teres major
triceps
latissimus dorsi
external oblique
gluteus medius
gluteus maximus
adductor magnus
vastus lateralis
gracilis
semitendinosus
biceps femoris
semimembranosus
gastrocnemius
Achilles tendon

Abductor Muscles (outer thigh/hip/buttock)

GLUTEUS MEDIUS

Origin – Outer surface of the ilium.
Insertion – Greater trochanter of the femur.
Action – Abduction of the hip.

GLUTEUS MINIMUS

Origin – Outer surface of the ilium (below medius attachment).
Insertion – Greater trochanter.
Action – Abduction of the hip.

TENSOR FASCIA LATAE

Origin – Anterior iliac crest.
Insertion – Via iliotibial band to lateral condyle of the femur, tibia and fibula.
Action – Abduction of the hip, assists with flexion of the hip.

Back of Lower Leg

GASTROCNEMIUS

Origin – Posterior condyles of the femur.
Insertion – Via the Achilles tendon to the calcaneus (heel bone).
Action – Plantar flexion of the ankle, assists with flexion of the knee.

SOLEUS

Origin – Upper posterior surfaces of the tibia and fibula.
Insertion – Via the Achilles tendon to the calcaneus (heel bone).
Action – Plantar flexion of the ankle.

Front of Lower Leg

ANTERIOR TIBIAL

Origin – Outer surface of the tibia.

Insertion – Medial cuneform of the tarsals of the foot and the first metatarsal.
Action – Dorsi-flexion of the ankle and inversion of the foot.

It should be noted that some muscles cross more than one joint. If a muscle crosses two joints it will influence both of them. With some muscles that cross two joints a paradoxical situation arises with certain movements. For example, one of the quadriceps muscles, rectus femoris, is involved in knee extension. Because it also crosses the hip joint, it is also involved in hip flexion. During actions such as walking, running and exercises such as lunging, the hip can be flexed at the same time as the knee is flexed. This can cause confusion within the muscle as inferior fibres will be involved in eccentric contraction (lengthening) and superior fibres in concentric contraction (shortening).

Likewise, the hamstring muscles cross both the back of the knee joint and the back of the hip joint. Hamstrings are involved in both knee flexion and hip extension. Again, during walking, running, lunging and squatting, the knee is flexed at the same time as the hip is flexed. Inferior fibres shorten while superior fibres lengthen. Because of this phenomenon, such muscles can be easily damaged, particularly in cases where there is an imbalance of strength between opposing muscles or there are tight muscles. Suppleness through stretching and strength through resistance training (including body weight) should be maintained.

It may have become clear from the above explanation that in order to identify the muscle being worked during a particular exercise we need to analyse the movement. If we first identify the joint or joints moving, and the type of joint movement, we can then identify which muscle causes that movement. That muscle will be the muscle worked during the positive phase of the exercise (body weight/resistance is moved against gravity). If a movement is with gravity, as is often the case during the negative/return phase of an exercise, then the muscle shortening may not necessarily be classed as a prime mover as it is not causing the movement (gravity is causing the movement). The muscle originally involved in concentric contraction and acting as a prime mover during the positive phase is now involved in eccentric contraction (lengthening) controlling the return. There are some schools of thought which class this as a prime mover, but I feel it is open to individual interpretation.

It should be clear that a good knowledge of the skeletal system, joint types and joint movements, muscle composition, contraction and action is essential for anyone involved in the performance, supervision or prescription of exercise.

3 Starting Positions, Posture, Stability and

There are four basic starting positions for exercises: standing, sitting, lying and kneeling. Those four basic starting positions can then be modified to give a variety of positions. Each modification of the basic starting position is given a name, but those names appear to be used

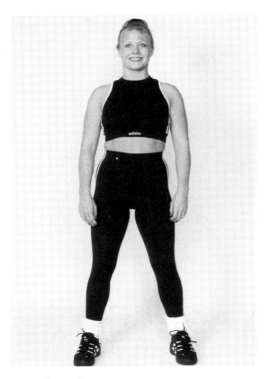

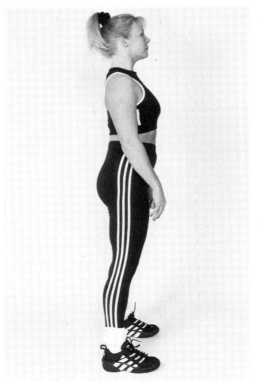

Fig. 14. The basic stance.

more in remedial exercise situations by professionals such as physiotherapists. Whatever name is given to the positions, or however they are described, such positions are adopted by all who exercise. Whatever the position, correct posture, stability and balance should be achieved in order to carry out the exercise safely and effectively.

STANDING POSITIONS

The basic stance for many free-standing exercises is achieved with the feet about shoulder-width apart, the knees slightly flexed (referred to as 'soft'). This helps position the pelvis so that the spine is in neutral alignment.

With the feet shoulder-width apart, a com-

paratively wide and stable base is achieved. Centre of gravity is approximately at the lower abdominal region and can easily be maintained over the base. This results in a stable position. Stability is important during free-standing exercises as loss of balance can cause sudden stretching movements and the risk of muscle tears. Severe loss of balance may result in a fall and associated consequences.

Having the knees slightly flexed or 'soft' not only protects the knee joints but also helps to position the pelvis and align the spine in a neutral position. Safe posture is maintained and balance encouraged. Good posture reduces negative tension in specific muscles and reduces stress on particular joints.

In the walk standing position, one foot is forward and the other back. Again, to assist with the maintenance of good posture and stability, the knees are kept soft and not locked out. This protects the knee joints and helps to achieve a neutral spine.

SITTING POSITIONS

In the long sitting position, the legs are outstretched, the knees extended and the hips are flexed so that the body is perpendicular at right angles to the legs.

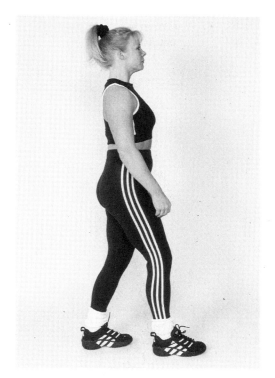

Fig. 15. Walk standing.

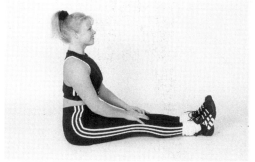

Fig. 16. Long sitting.

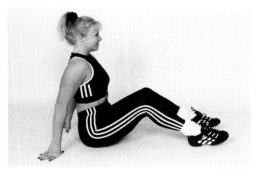

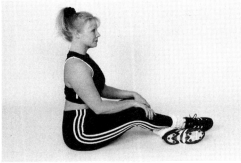

Fig. 17. Crook sitting.

This position is often adopted as the starting position for a number of exercises such as seated hamstring stretch, or to perform remedial exercises for the quadriceps by tensing the quads and slightly lifting the straight leg. However, by sitting with two straight legs there is an amount of stress imposed upon the lumbar spine, and care must be taken if an exercise then involves further forward flexion of the hips or forward flexion of the spine. The stress can be relieved to some degree by flexing one knee (and therefore one hip) so that only one leg is straight.

Crook sitting is a sitting position with the knees flexed and the feet on the floor. This can be a comfortable position with reduced stress on the lumbar spine because the hip flexor muscles are no longer stretched and no longer pull as tightly on the lumbar vertebrae.

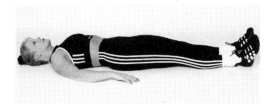

Fig. 18. Supine lying.

LYING POSITIONS

The supine lying position is lying face-up with the legs straight. This position may be the basis for a total body stretch, but even this position imposes some stress on the lumbar spine because the hip flexor muscles are stretched and develop powerful stretch tension which pulls the lumbar spine into hyperextension (lordosis: the lower back will curve upwards so that an arch is formed upwards from the floor).

Crook lying is a supine position (face up) but with the knees flexed and the feet on the floor – a very comfortable position, and a very good one for the relief of lower back pain. Also, it is the recommended start position for the majority of abdominal exercises. With the knees flexed, the hip flexors are passively shortened and exert very little pull on the lumbar spine. In this position, the lower back will be down against the floor.

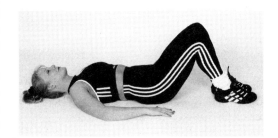

Fig. 19. Crook lying.

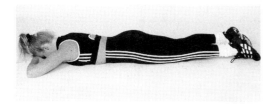

Fig. 20. Prone lying.

Basically, prone lying is lying face down with the legs straight, but this position can be modified by the position of the arms which may be down by the sides, level with the chest (as if starting a press-up), by the side of the head, or even stretched out beyond the head. With exercises such as trunk raises to strengthen the back, the position of the arms will affect leverage and therefore the resistance.

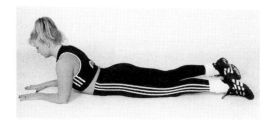

Fig. 21. Forearm support prone lying.

In the prone-lying position the arms may be placed under the chest to support the upper body so that the spine is passively extended. This position may be referred to as forearm support prone lying.

The side-lying position is lying on the side, usually with the head resting on a flexed arm, or with the elbow resting on the floor and the head supported in the hand and by the arm. Often the knees are kept soft. If the intention is to work the abductor muscles of the uppermost side, then

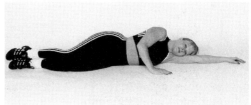

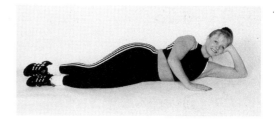

Fig. 22. Side lying.

the pelvis must be pushed slightly forwards and the body weight allowed to roll slightly forwards, supported by the hand placed on the floor in front of the body.

KNEELING POSITIONS

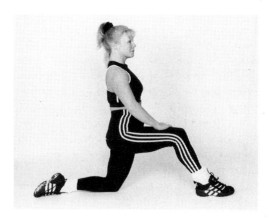

Fig. 23. Half kneeling.

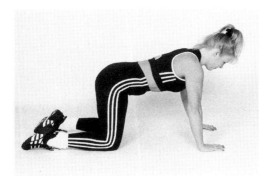

Fig. 24. Prone kneeling.

In half kneeling, one knee is flexed and resting on the floor. The other knee is flexed but the foot is on the floor. Ensure that the back is held upright and not stooping forwards.

The prone kneeling position is sometimes referred to as the 'box' position. Both knees are flexed and resting on the floor. The shins are parallel to the floor and the thighs at ninety degrees and perpendicular. The back is parallel to the floor, the hands on the floor with the arms supporting the upper body. This is the start position for the 'box' press-up and for hip extensions to strengthen and tone the gluteals (hip extensors).

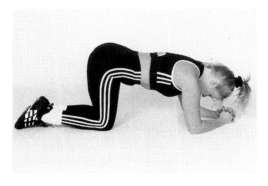

Fig. 25. Inclined prone kneeling.

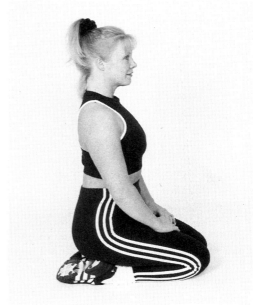

Fig. 26. Kneel sitting.

Inclined prone kneeling involves adopting a prone kneeling position and then lowering the upper body down towards the floor. The weight of the upper body can then be supported by the flexed arms with the forearms resting on the floor. This is a variation of the 'box' position and may be a comfortable position for hip extensions.

The kneel-sitting position involves kneeling and then lowering the seat down towards, or to rest upon, the heels. This may be a comfortable position for some people and a very relaxing one, but for others there is the danger of stressing the knee joint by 'forcing it open' as a result of hyperflexion under the weight of the upper body.

The kneel-sitting position could be adopted to stretch the muscles at the front of the lower leg, although it is recommended that some of the body weight is supported by the arms held down by the sides and the hands/fingers touching the floor.

Unfortunately, also from this position a person might attempt the particularly hazardous and not recommended manoeuvre of leaning backwards with the intention of stretching the quadriceps at the front of the thigh.

With any kneeling position it is recommended that the kneecaps do not form the base in contact with the floor and upon which the weight is borne. This would be painful and uncomfortable at the time, but may also lead to other long-term conditions of the patella and its underlying cartilage.

Whatever exercise is to be performed, and whatever starting position is adopted, it is important to ensure that good posture, stability and balance are achieved and maintained throughout. In the position adopted, joints should be correctly aligned so that excessive and unnatural stresses are not imposed on muscles and joints. The centre of gravity should always remain over the base. The wider the base, the more stable is an object (and the body). It is not recommended, however, that in a standing position a very wide base is formed with the feet and the knees locked straight. The weight of the body will press vertically downwards and can impose stress to the medial (inner) aspect of the knee joints. Nor is it recommended that performers stand with the feet close together. This will create a narrow base and an unstable position.

Exercises involve movement and a shifting of body weight. We should endeavour to be in control of that body weight and maintain positions whereby the weight remains over the base and we are stable and in balance. Large swinging movements can develop momentum, a force which continues the movement in a certain direction. Care should be taken as momentum can adversely affect stability and balance. All movements should be controlled.

4 Warm-Up and Cool-Down

It is vitally important to perform a warm-up before and a cool-down after every exercise/training session. The body is very similar to a motor car's engine which takes time to reach an optimum working temperature. The body, too, cannot perform to its full potential if cold, and cannot cope as effectively with the stresses of training or competition.

WARM-UP

The warm-up is carried out at an intensity well below that anticipated for the actual training session. It should start off at a very low intensity and gradually progress, yet not reach too high an intensity that it becomes a training session in itself. In general, a warm-up, before any type of physical activity, should consist of three components:

1. *Mobilizers* – gentle movements of a number of joints to loosen and lubricate the joint.

2. *Pulse raisers* – movements, usually involving travel from the spot, which increase respiration and heart rate.

3. *Stretches* – gentle stretches held for about 7 to 10 seconds to loosen and relax the muscles.

Mobilizers and pulse raisers do not need to be separate, individual components, but can be integrated into one general activity. Imaginative exercise teachers can have their charges move about and include a multitude of joint movements simultaneously. However, the *stretches should always be performed as the last part of the warm-up after the muscles have been warmed* by gentle movement (Rosenbaum and Henning, 1995). It is *not* recommended that cold muscles are stretched, yet unfortunately so many people start off their warm-up with stretches.

The warm-up prepares the body gradually for the intensity of the activity to follow and has two potential benefits: it should *enhance the performance* to follow (whether a training session or competition) and *reduce the risk of injury*.

A number of physiological changes occur in the body during and as a result of the warm-up:

1. Heart rate increases.

2. Cardiac output increases.

3. Respiration increases.

4. Blood supply to the working muscles is increased.

These four factors result in an increase in nutrients and oxygen to the working muscles.

5. The aerobic energy system is given time to come into effective operation.

6. Muscles are warmed, stretched and loosened.

7. Joints are warmed, loosened and lubricated. (The movement stimulates the flow of synovial fluid into the joint.)

8. The secretion of adrenaline is increased to speed up metabolism.

Before a sporting competition, a fourth part of

the warm-up – skills practice – will often be performed.

Skills practice will include practice of all the skills to be performed in the game and will help develop/confirm confidence in those skills, allow opportunity to adjust to lighting, surroundings, court conditions, observe the ability of the opposition and so on. For example, the 'knock-up' in squash, badminton or tennis; the 'kick about' before a football match; running, hitting, stopping, etc, before hockey; throwing, catching and batting before cricket. These activities should not form the warm-up in themselves but should be performed *after* a full physical warm-up has been performed.

A correct warm-up can decrease the stress on the heart. Performing a vigorous activity without a warm-up can result in the heart muscle not receiving enough oxygen. Warming up will lower blood pressure and increase blood flow to the heart (Stamford, 1995a).

COOL-DOWN

A cool-down should be carried out at the end of the training session or immediately after competition. The cool-down will consist of a continuation of activity at a reduced intensity and stretching of the muscles that have been worked.

The cool-down allows the systems of the body that have been working very hard to return gradually towards normal. It will assist with a speedier removal of waste products from the muscles and bloodstream and it maintains circulation, particularly the return of venous blood to the heart. Cool-down helps to lower the levels of adrenaline produced during exercise. Adrenaline which stays in the bloodstream while at rest can stress the heart (Stamford, 1995a).

During exercise, two responses occur: blood pressure rises and adrenal substances (adrenaline [epinephrine] and norepinephrine) are secreted into the bloodstream. After exercise blood pressure falls, but the adrenal substances continue to rise, stimulating the heart to beat fast but inefficiently. Blood pools in the legs and does not return easily to the heart. This can result in an inadequate blood supply to the tissues of the heart muscle and result in cardiac trauma (Cooper, 1980, 1986).

While we are active, circulation is maintained by the pumping action of the working muscles, particularly those of the lower limbs. A lot of blood is in the lower limbs and has to be forced upwards against gravity. The heart cannot cope with that task on its own and relies on the additional pumping action of the muscles. If we were to stop suddenly at the end of a vigorous activity the muscular pumping action would cease and blood would tend to pool in the lower limbs. As insufficient blood is getting back to the heart, and therefore insufficient oxygenated blood is being circulated to the brain, lightheadedness and fainting can occur.

In addition, the heart tries harder to maintain circulation and may beat even faster. Consequently, extra stress is placed on an already hard-working heart (how many cases of heart trauma occur *after* vigorous exercise rather than *during*?!). A potentially dangerous, even life-threatening, situation arises if we stop suddenly after vigorous exercise.

After a period of reduced-intensity activity, a series of brief stretches should be carried out as part of the cool-down. Stretches, which may now be held for longer than 7 to 10 seconds while the muscles are warm, loosen the muscles which have just been contracted and help to develop and maintain their suppleness and elasticity, contributing to the flexibility of the joints.

5 The Involvement and Effect of Levers and Leverage

LEVERS

A lever employs a rigid bar (lever arm), a pivot point (fulcrum: F) and an effort source (effort: E)

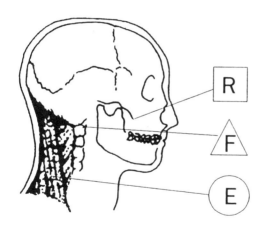

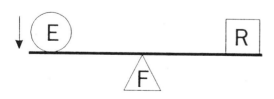

Fig. 27. A first-class lever.

to overcome a resistance (R). Leverage is the application of a force to overcome a resistance using a rigid bar, a pivot point and an effort source.

Levers are employed in the body and every move we make involves leverage. The bones are the rigid bars, the moveable joints are the pivot points and the muscles provide the effort.

There are three types (or classes) of lever and all three are employed in the body.

A first-class lever. In the body, a good example is the skull which pivots on the atlas vertebra at the top of the neck. The weight of the skull can tilt it forwards (resistance); the joint between the base of the skull and the atlas vertebra is the fulcrum, and the muscles at the back of the neck provide the effort to tilt it backwards.

A second-class lever. An example in the body is when we rise up on to our toes. The ball of the foot in contact with the floor is the pivot point; the resistance is the body weight pressing down through the ankle, and the effort is from the calf muscles which lift up the heel bone. The rigid bar is the length of the foot, which is made rigid by the fixing action of other muscles.

A third-class lever. There are many examples in the body, but an obvious example is when the elbow is flexed. The forearm is the rigid bar; the resistance is the weight of the forearm and hand

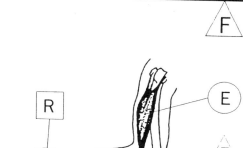

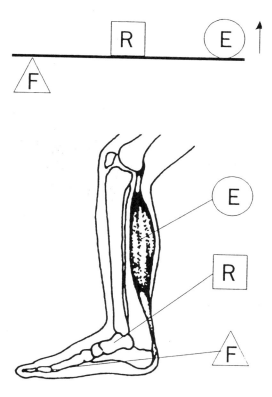

Fig. 28. A second-class lever.

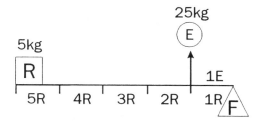

Fig. 29. A third-class lever.

and any additional weight which may be held in the hand. The elbow joint is the pivot point, and the effort is provided by the biceps muscle.

The third-class lever is the most common lever in the body. It is actually an inefficient lever because in most cases it involves a very short effort arm (the distance from the muscle attachment to the joint) and a very long resistance arm (the distance from the resistance to the joint). However, this particular lever, though inefficient in overcoming resistances, is employed in the body to create great range and speed of movement. A small amount of movement from the effort muscle will create a large

amount of movement at the end of a limb. As for overcoming resistances, skeletal muscles usually have enough strength to develop huge forces to overcome heavy resistances.

The law of levers dictates that the resistance is multiplied by the length of the resistance arm, and if we apply an effort to overcome that resistance it will have to overcome that resulting resistance. If the resistance was 5kg and the resistance arm was five times the length of the effort arm, we would require 5 x 5kg (25kg) in effort to overcome that resistance.

Fig. 30. A third-class lever illustrating the law of levers.

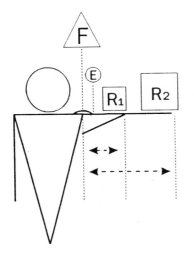

Fig. 31. Vertical abduction of the shoulder.

EFFECTS OF LEVERS

The law of levers and leverage has important implications for exercises. When moving a body part against gravity, or lifting an additional weight, a long resistance arm will have the effect of increasing that weight and therefore require a greater force from the effort muscle. In some people that muscle may not be strong enough to cope. Also, if the lever arm is long because a joint part-way along it is fixed by other muscles, then the extreme resistance may place stress on that joint or on the muscles attempting to fix it. For example, the elbow is fixed when lifting a straight arm sideways (vertical abduction).

One very important application of a third-class lever in the body involves hip flexion and

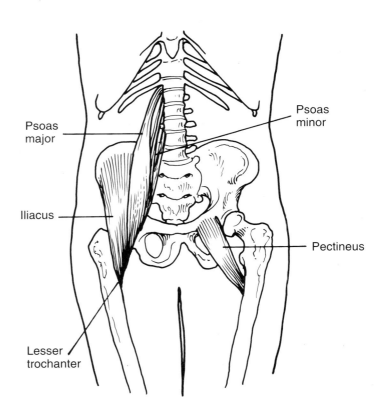

Fig. 32. The hip flexor muscle.

the hip flexor muscles. The hip flexor muscles consist of the psoas and iliacus which are collectively referred to as ilio-psoas. They are deep muscles, not necessarily obvious to persons lacking a knowledge of anatomy.

Iliacus has its origin of attachment on the inside of the crest of the ilium, whereas psoas has its origin on the twelfth thoracic vertebra and all the lumbar vertebrae and sacrum. The two muscles combine to form one common insertion attachment on the lesser trochanter of the femur (inner side of the thigh bone) and they are duplicated on either side of the spine.

As their name suggests, the main purpose of the hip flexor muscles is to flex the hip joint, lifting up the thigh, but if the legs are fixed, they will pull the trunk forwards or upwards (depending on the body's position), which is also flexion of the hip joint.

The fact that the lumbar vertebrae are involved is particularly important. It should be appreciated that the origin of attachment is not a solid or rigid bone, but a flexible column of irregular bones. If a person were to lie on his/her back with the legs extended, the hip flexor muscles are stretched and consequently there is a pull on both attachment points. As the origin (the lumbar spine) is flexible, this pull results in a curve of the lumbar spine, which is pulled into hyperextension.

To attempt to lift two straight legs from this position would involve the hip flexor muscles

having to work against a very long lever, generate a very high tension, and create excessive pull on the lumbar spine, causing further hyperextension, stretching of the abdominal muscles and an increase in intra-abdominal pressure, all presenting a potentially dangerous situation (Mitchell and Dale, 1980).

Many people believe this exercise is for strengthening the abdominal muscles, but the main muscles involved are the hip flexors. The abdominals only act as fixators, tensing to brace the trunk and hold an isometric contraction which can result in an increase in blood pressure. In addition, most people instinctively hold their breath, which greatly increases abdominal pressure and can be dangerous.

Likewise, when performing a full sit-up, the feet may be anchored and the movement requires hip flexion and so the hip flexor muscles are the main muscles involved. Again, these have to work against a long and heavy lever and exert a very strong pulling force on the lumbar spine. The abdominals tense into isometric contraction to brace the trunk, but persons with abdominal weakness may allow the trunk to extend which stretches the abdominal muscles.

It should be obvious therefore that the two exercises mentioned above, straight leg raises and full sit-ups, could be considered controversial or contra-indicated as they do not necessarily achieve what the performer wants to achieve, they work muscles against long levers

Fig. 33. Leverage involved in straight leg lifts (dangerous).

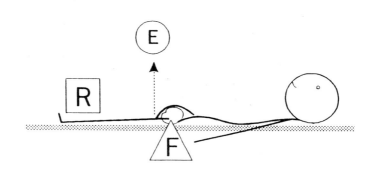

and very heavy resistances, and are potentially dangerous for the lower back (for safer and more effective abdominal exercises, see Chapter 9, Abdominal Exercises).

CHANGE OF LEVERAGE

Other exercises can be made easier or harder by altering the leverage. In the mechanical world, we would probably lengthen the effort arm of a lever to make the work easier. In the body, the length of the effort arm is determined by the muscle attachment, which we cannot alter. We can, however, in many cases alter the length of the resistance arm. This is done by flexing a limb (shortening the lever [resistance arm]) or extending a limb (lengthening the lever [resistance arm]), as with vertical abduction of the shoulder already mentioned.

Reverse leg raises to work the gluteal muscles can be progressed or adapted by altering the length of the lever. In the 'box' position (kneeling, but for this exercise with elbows resting on the floor), the hip is extended by lifting one thigh backwards and upwards. With the knee flexed, the lever is short and the resistance reduced. With the knee extended, the lever is lengthened and the resistance increased.

NB. We may consider the involvement of the hamstrings during the reverse leg raises. As the hamstrings cross the hip joint they will be involved as synergists during hip extension. With the knee flexed, which produces a short lever and therefore less resistance, the involvement of the hamstrings is reduced. It might be considered that gluteus maximus (the prime mover in hip extension) has to work harder because it is not assisted by the hamstrings. However, in practice, it will be felt that the exercise is harder with an extended knee (long lever). I feel that even though the hamstrings may now be more involved, the longer lever and increased resistance works gluteus maximus harder.

Lateral leg raises to work the hip abductor muscles can also be made easier or harder by altering the leverage. The uppermost leg is lifted vertically/laterally either with a flexed knee

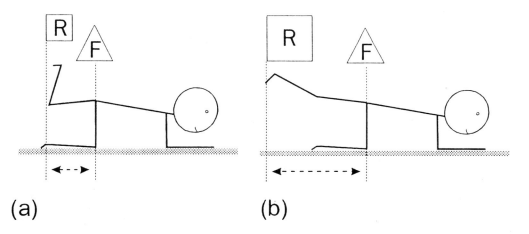

(a)   (b)

Fig. 34. Reverse leg raises performed against (a) a short lever; (b) a long lever.

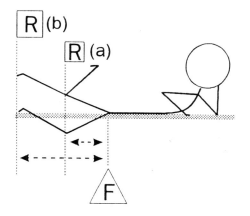

Fig. 35. Lateral leg raises performed against (a) a short lever; (b) a long lever.

(short lever/light resistance) or an extended knee (long lever/heavier resistance).

Abdominal curls performed on the floor can be carried out with the hands resting on the thighs to create the effect of a short lever, as some of the body weight is placed nearer to the fulcrum (pivot point) and away from the end of the resistance arm. Performed with the arms across the chest it has a similar effect to increasing the lever slightly, as some of the weight is moved away from the fulcrum part-way along the resistance arm, which increases the resistance. With the hands by the side of the head, weight is transferred to the end of the resistance arm thus increasing the resistance further.

In the three progressions of abdominal curl, resistance is increased by moving weight away from the pivot point and along the resistance arm: (a) easy, (b) moderate, (c) hard (see Chapter 9).

Back/trunk raises to strengthen the extensor muscles of the spine can likewise be made easier or harder by moving weight along the lever arm. The exercise involves lying prone and raising the upper body in a controlled manner with the legs

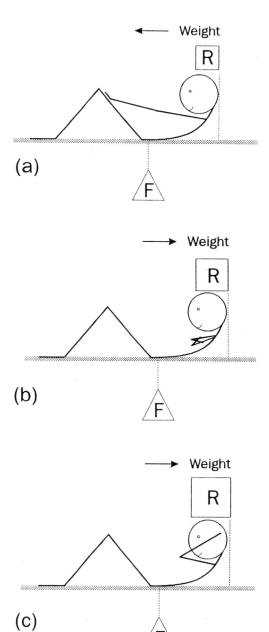

Fig. 36. Three progressions of abdominal curl.

Fig. 37. Full trunk hyperextensions: dangerous and not recommended.

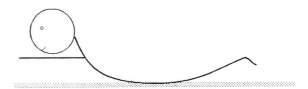

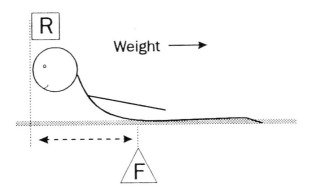

Fig. 38. Trunk raises employing the effect of a short lever (easy).

Fig. 39. Trunk raises employing the effect of a longer lever (harder).

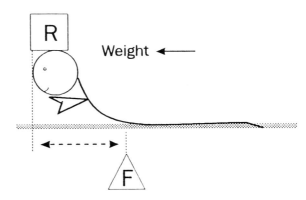

remaining on the floor. However, this should not be performed as a ballistic hyperextension, as has traditionally been practised by a number of sports people.

With the arms placed by the sides, some of the body weight is transferred closer to the pivot point, thus reducing the resistance (see fig. 38).

With the hands placed by the side of the head or under the chin, body weight is transferred towards the end of the resistance arm and the resistance is increased (see fig. 39).

If the arms were held out forwards beyond the head, the resistance arm would be lengthened considerably and the resistance would be increased.

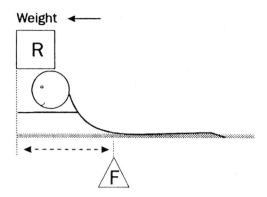

Fig. 40. Trunk raises employing a long lever (hard).

NB The above-mentioned extensions of the spine performed to strengthen the back should be carried out with great care. There should be no fast jerking; there is no need to lift into extreme hyperextension; the upper chest and shoulders need only be lifted a couple of inches (5 cm) off the floor; and the head should not be lifted back, which would mean hyperextending the neck.

The resistance during a press-up exercise can be altered by reducing or increasing the lever.

The box press-up (fig. 41), (a) involves a short lever (short resistance arm) and is therefore comparatively easy. The three-quarter press-up (b) involves a longer lever and is therefore harder. The full press-up (c) involves an even longer lever and is therefore harder still.

CHANGE OF LEVERAGE WITH JOINT ANGLE

It is the *horizontal* distance from the pivot point to the end of the lever arm that influences the

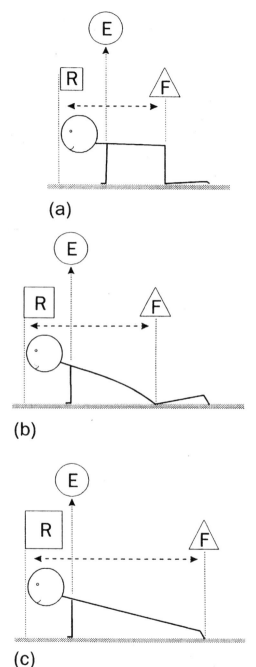

Fig. 41. Progressions of press-up.

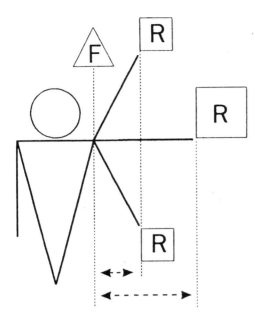

Fig. 42. Change of horizontal distance.

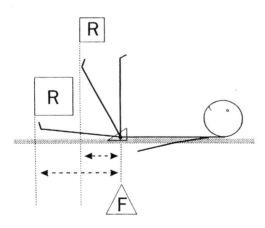

Fig. 43. Reduction in
length of the lever
arm as the legs come
towards the vertical.

resistance. Therefore, a limb or body part is heaviest when in a horizontal position and parallel to the floor. At a different joint angle, the resistance will decrease because the horizontal distance is reduced.

A greater effort is required from the deltoid (Fig. 42) when the arm is horizontal than when it is at an angle because of the change in horizontal distance from the shoulder joint (fulcrum/pivot point) to the end of the arm.

Holding two straight legs in a position lifted from the floor when lying supine can be very dangerous and can impose tremendous stress upon the lumbar spine. This is because the hip flexor muscles have to exert a very high force against a long lever. The horizontal distance from the hip joint to the end of the limb is great and therefore the resistance high. If the legs are moved to a vertical position, which may be adopted in certain abdominal exercises, the horizontal distance is greatly reduced and the pull of the hip flexor muscles is therefore eliminated.

It will have become obvious from the previous information that a knowledge of the body is required when performing exercises. To be more precise, a knowledge of kinesiology – the study of movement – is required. During exercise, we need to know which joints are moving and which muscles are causing or controlling the movement. We may also need to know which joints are fixed and which muscles are fixing them.

In addition, we have to have some knowledge of mechanics. Unless we understand about levers and leverage, how the resistance can be influenced by leverage, and how we can alter the leverage, we cannot necessarily perform safe and effective exercise.

6 Controversial and Contra-indicated Exercises

'Controversial' means 'open to controversy'; 'Controversy' means 'disputation' (*Oxford English Dictionary*). Dispute or discussion concerning some exercises focuses on whether or not they are safe and effective. As a result of scientific study, some traditionally practised exercises are now considered by the majority of knowledgeable and qualified professionals as being potentially dangerous. If we have a knowledge of how the body works, consider what effect the exercise is *supposed* to have, and what effect the exercise *actually* has, we find that some exercises are better left well alone by the majority of people.

'Contra-indicated' in scientific and medical circles means 'not recommended', 'dangerous', 'not achieving the desired results', and with reference to exercise suggests that certain exercises require the body to produce movements or adopt positions for which it was not designed.

For example, a joint may have a great range of movement from fully flexed to fully extended, but it is not designed to go beyond that full extension into hyperextension. Some joints may be damaged by repetitive hyperflexion under weight-bearing load (e.g. the knee). Some exercises attempt to take joints beyond their normal full range. Also, muscles are designed to contract against resistances and to lengthen, sometimes while trying to hold back against a resistance (eccentric contraction). The muscle will lengthen to its maximum. To ballistically bounce that muscle will develop tension and may tear muscle fibres and connective tissue which were not designed to be vigorously and powerfully stretched by a repetitive external force.

Generally speaking, controversial and contra-indicated exercises are more or less one and the same thing, even though we can differentiate. Many exercises are controversial *because* they are contra-indicated: either they are not appropriate for the body part, or do not achieve what the individual requires.

But we have to put exercises into perspective. Some exercises may generally be regarded as having a high degree of risk, but in some instances may be indicated (necessary) because of a particular person's sport or profession. For example, dancers, gymnasts, some power athletes and participants in the combat sports may carry out ballistic bounce stretches, achieve extreme positions, hold powerful isometric contractions, hyperflex joints under body weight, or perform very high repetitions of high-intensity movements. However, such are the demands of their chosen sport or occupation that they have to train their bodies to cope with such stresses. The sports person or dancer has chosen that particular activity, may have ambitions for top competition or championship glory, and accepts the risks involved in the training as well as in the competition. Furthermore, that person's competitive career at that level is likely to be comparatively short-term as the natural effects of ageing, and the rigours of high-intensity training will take their toll. Again, the sports person, dancer, gymnast must be prepared to accept that fact.

This does not mean that all sports persons and athletes can carry out any exercise, whatever the risk. Far from it. For many of the exercises with a high risk there are alternative exercises which have less risk and may be more effective. A knowledgeable and wise athlete will carry out the safer and more effective exercise.

It could be suggested that almost every exercise carries some degree of risk. There may be more risk for one person than another. Ability, fitness level, natural flexibility, natural strength and so on will influence how much risk there is. Cullum and Mowbray (1989) stated that not every exercise can be performed by all individuals. Different body types provide natural obstacles for some exercises and this is often overlooked by performers, teachers and coaches. Almost every exercise can be harmful if done incorrectly.

Many people are exercising for health-related reasons (health-related fitness). For them, it is hoped that exercise will be carried out, enjoyed and will remain safe and effective well into older age − a way of life. For those people, exercises need to be safe and effective and the high intensities and extreme positions practised by some elite performers are definitely contra-indicated. The 'no pain, no gain' philosophy is totally inappropriate for the majority of people. A well-chosen and well-performed exercise will always be accompanied by a sense of satisfaction and pleasure, and although it may be hard work there will never be any sense of strain (Mitchell and Dale, 1980).

We have to ask ourselves what is the purpose of our training, or what is the purpose of a particular exercise. Obviously, we want to achieve maximum benefit at minimum risk. If by performing a particular exercise the potential dangers outweigh the benefits, then that exercise is controversial/contra-indicated. Some exercises may not appear unsafe because we do not necessarily feel pain or strain while performing them. In addition, we may have been performing a particular exercise in a particular way for years and have not had any trouble. That exercise may still be contra-indicated as the damage being done through long-term repetition is on a microscopic scale (micro-trauma) and may take quite a long time to manifest. Examples include forward bending with straight legs, trunk rotations while bending forwards with straight legs, vigorous trunk rotations using the momentum of a broom handle or bar across the shoulders, straight-leg raises, straight-leg sit-ups, over-zealous side bends, hyperextensions of the spine, all of which can cause micro-trauma to the inter-vertebral discs and vertebral joints.

Any person involved in exercise and training needs to have a good working knowledge of anatomy (the structure of the body), physiology (the function of the body) and kinesiology (the science of movement and how the body moves), and leverage. Without this knowledge, how can a person know whether or not an exercise is safe or effective?

Certain illnesses and conditions provide contra-indications to exercise and training. It is sometimes claimed that a simple head cold, although unpleasant, need not stop training. In fact, some may claim that exercising during a cold infection may actually make a person feel better, but others choose to rest up for a few days.

More severe viral infections, on the other hand, such as influenza and respiratory tract infections (RTI), particularly of the chest, are more serious and we should not try to train with a virus. The body needs all its strength to fight off the virus and training can weaken the body and suppress the immune system.

Symptoms of a respiratory tract infection may

worsen after exercise. Often there is inflammation of the airways and increased bronchial secretions. In individuals with asthma or reactive airways caused by RTI, strenuous exercise may cause bronchiospasm. Certain viral infections can lead to splenic rupture or myocarditis (inflammation of the heart muscle). Also some infections may reduce muscle strength and fluid levels in the body (Primos, 1996; Cooper, 1986).

EXERCISE ADDICTION AND OBSESSION

Some people become addicted to exercise. The athlete or sports person in serious competition may need to train every day and in some cases, twice a day. However, this is not the case for those exercising for health-related fitness, and they will certainly not be doing the same type of exercise.

The American College of Sports Medicine (ACSM), advising on exercise in general for the development and maintenance of cardio-respiratory fitness, body composition and muscular strength and endurance, recommends the following:

Frequency: 3–5 days per week.

Intensity: 60–90% of maximum heart rate.

Duration: 20–60 minutes of continuous aerobic activity.

Mode: Any activity that uses large muscle groups, can be maintained continuously and is rhythmical and aerobic in nature.

Resistance/Strength training: Moderate intensity, one set of 8–12 repetitions of 8–10 exercises involving the major muscle groups at least two days per week.

Although exercise should be performed regularly, strengthening and toning exercises should not necessarily be performed on the same muscle groups on consecutive days, and the need for rest and recovery as part of an exercise or training programme should be realized. This fact is not always recognized by serious athletes and fatigue, over-training and injury result.

De Mond (1993) spoke of both the *quantity* and *quality* of exercise needed to be fit in an injury-free fashion, and of the difference between exercising for health-related benefits and exercising for fitness. Also Bouchart *et al.* (1993) claimed the stimulus to promote health probably differs from that required to increase fitness.

I have used the term 'health-related fitness' to suggest we desire a level of fitness which promotes a healthy state in the body. Moderation, as always, is perhaps the key word. Excesses of anything are usually detrimental. The need for daily doses of high-intensity exercise is a recipe for disaster, but some people still believe in the 'no pain, no gain' philosophy.

Although exercise should become a part of everyday life, it should not dominate it. When the need for exercise supersedes everything else in day-to-day life, one has become addicted and obsessive.

However, addiction to exercise may not necessarily be a bad thing in itself. There are worse addictions, such as smoking, alcohol, drugs, etc. Crisp (1997) suggested that the benefits that do exist, even with obsessive exercise regimes, possibly outweigh the risks.

Crisp suggested that exercise, in the form of addiction, is perhaps a *symptom* and not a *cause*. With some people there may be the need for a daily 'fix' of endorphins. This chemical is the body's natural anti-depressant and painkiller – nature's 'Prozac' and 'Brufen' rolled into one. The feelings during and after exercise can certainly be pleasurable, but would that indicate addiction?

In most cases the cause is psychological with exercise the *manifestation*. Obsession with weight and body composition may be a borderline case of anorexia nervosa or bulimia. Job-related stress may cause some to 'hit the bottle', whereas for others the gym is daily solace. In both these cases, the problem is not with exercise in itself but with other factors which need to be recognized and treated.

So the problem is not necessarily with exercise *per se*, but with the effect it may have on everyday life, on marriage, partners, family, friends, work and social life. Exercise addiction and obsession can become a problem, but the biggest problem for the majority of the population is not exercising enough. For that small minority who may become addicted, try to recognize the fact, and determine why. Treat the cause and the symptom will be controlled.

Part Two: Strengthening and Toning

7 Introduction to Strengthening and Toning

Strengthening and toning involves working muscles regularly against varying amounts of resistance. Hypertrophy of the muscle occurs, which results in a stronger muscle. The exercises in this section employ body weight, gravity and leverage to create that resistance. Training with weights is a separate, specialist topic and is not covered within the pages of this book. Working muscles regularly against resistances will increase and maintain muscle strength, increase and maintain muscle tone, and develop muscular endurance.

Strength is defined as the ability for a muscle or muscles to exert maximal force to overcome a resistance. The strength of a muscle is proportional to its cross-sectional size and therefore if the muscle increases in size (hypertrophy), it increases in strength. However, this does not mean that we have to body-build in order to increase strength. Significant increases in

strength can occur with minimal enlargement of the muscle.

Muscle tone is a healthy condition of the muscle and its connection with the nervous system; the muscle is in a state of continuous stimulation and semi-contraction, ready to work. Tone is a necessary quality in the postural muscles, which have to maintain degrees of continual contraction.

Muscular endurance is the ability for muscles to perform a higher number of contractions against lighter/moderate resistances. Low resistance/high repetition training increases the ability of the muscle to take up and process oxygen.

In order to carry out strengthening and toning exercises safely and effectively, a knowledge of the structure and function of the body is necessary to ensure (a) that the exercise works the desired muscle, and (b) that the body is not subjected to unnatural stresses which could result in injury.

Chapters 3 and 5 are of particular importance regarding starting positions, posture, stability, balance and leverage.

Another important safety consideration when performing strengthening and toning exercises is *breathing*. With the majority of strengthening and toning exercises it is recommended that performers breathe *out* on the *effort* (the positive phase) and *in* on the *return* (the negative phase). Breathing should also be comparatively explosive and rhythmical, and the breath should never be held. Holding the breath during muscular contractions increases blood pressure, increases intra-abdominal pressure, reduces blood flow back to the heart and to the brain, and therefore creates considerable risk. With abdominal exercises in particular it is important not to hold the breath, and to exhale on the effort and inhale on the return.

With strengthening and toning exercises, resistance can be influenced by body position. Changes in body position can involve or eliminate the effect of gravity to increase or decrease resistance, or can alter the leverage to increase or decrease resistance (see Chapter 5, 'The Involvement and Effect of Levers and Leverage').

GRAVITY

Gravity is the force that pulls objects towards the surface of the earth and is responsible for weight. Our body weight, either as a whole, or the weight of part of the body, acts as a resistance which muscles must work to overcome.

Muscles work (contract) to move joints, and if they contract to lift weight against the force of gravity they work harder. Very often a muscle can be made to work to move a joint but with very little resistance and therefore with little

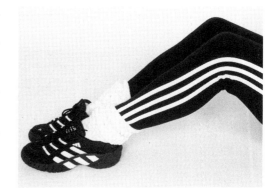

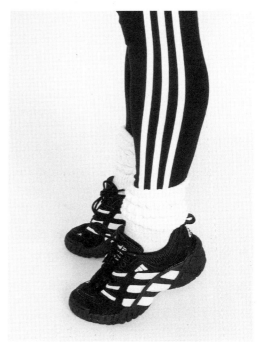

Fig. 44. Working the muscles of the calf.

force. If we alter our body position, that same muscle may then be required to move that same joint, but now to do so the muscle must overcome gravity and lift body weight.

For example, if the body is in a long sitting

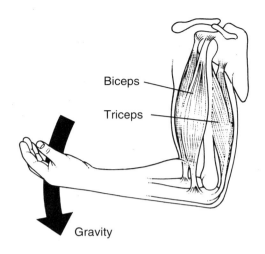

Fig. 45. Return of a biceps curl.

position, the muscles of the calf (gastrocnemius and soleus) can be contracted to move the ankle joint (plantar flexion). If we simply stand up and create the same movement, which would lift us up onto our toes, the muscles of the calf have to create a higher force to lift the body weight.

If the knee is flexed with the body in a side-lying position the hamstrings will contract to cause that movement. If we roll into a prone-lying position and the knee is flexed, the hamstrings have to work harder against gravity

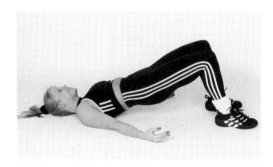

Fig. 47. Crook lying position to work the extensors of the spine and the gluteals.

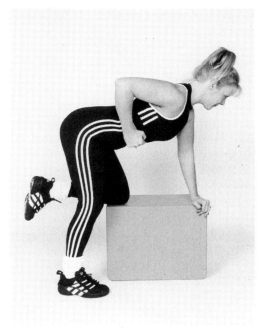

Fig. 46. Supported bent-over position.

to lift the weight of the lower leg.

With most strengthening and toning exercises, in order to be working against gravity, the muscle must be facing upwards and the body would have to be positioned accordingly to cause that muscle to face upwards.

For example, although the return phase of a biceps curl involves elbow extension, the triceps is not worked because movement occurs in the direction of, and therefore with, gravity. To work the triceps we would have to position the body so that the triceps faces upwards to extend the elbow against gravity.

In the return of a biceps curl, gravity causes the downward movement, not the triceps.

In a supported bent-over position, the upper arm is placed so that the triceps faces upwards and can work against gravity.

Exceptions to having the triceps face upwards

51

can occur when using resistance equipment with pulleys. The working muscle may be facing downwards, but the weight stack (resistance) moves upwards against gravity.

Another exception to this rule would be when achieving a crook-lying position to work the extensor muscles of the spine and the gluteals. Some people may believe this works the 'lower' abdominals because the pelvis is lifted up. However, the pelvis is not pulled upwards by the abdominals, but is pushed upwards as the lower back and hips are extended. In fact, the abdominals are lengthened. Obviously, the extensors of the spine and the gluteals in this case are facing downwards.

LEVERAGE

By producing a movement with a limb held in a bent (flexed) position, the resistance is low because the lever is short. If the limb is held in a straight (extended) position, the resistance is increased because the lever is lengthened. Most movements involve muscles, bones and joints forming a third-class lever (see Chapter 5, 'The Influence and Effect of Levers and Leverage').

By bending a limb we reduce the resistance arm of the lever, and by straightening a limb we increase the resistance arm of the lever. The amount of effort required from the muscle to overcome the resistance is equivalent to that resistance multiplied by the horizontal length of the lever (from the pivot point to the end of the lever arm).

A BALANCED PROGRAMME

It is important with strengthening and toning exercises to carry out a balanced programme; opposing muscles should be worked within an exercise programme. Any movement requires two muscles to work together: one will shorten to cause the movement and the other will lengthen to control the movement. The muscle which shortens to cause the movement is known as the *prime mover*, and the muscle which lengthens to control the movement is known as the *antagonist*. The two muscles working together are known as *antagonistic pairs*, or *opposing muscles*. If one muscle is worked as a prime mover, then at some stage in the exercise programme the opposing muscle should also be worked as a prime mover.

Exercise movements should not be rushed. They should be carried out with a controlled movement, especially on the return or negative phase. The muscle which has just acted as a prime mover, shortening to cause the movement, was involved in *concentric* contraction. On the return it is involved in *eccentric* contraction. Eccentric contraction involves the muscle fibres trying to hold back against the resistance and 'paying out'. Fast, ballistic-type movements will invoke a strong stretch reflex in the muscle which will result in an increase in tension. A fast, uncontrolled movement can build up momentum which will tug at and forcefully lengthen the muscle fibres which are trying to contract. The recommended technique for safe and effective strengthening and toning exercises involves slower, controlled movements.

Held contractions are not recommended either, especially against an increased resistance, such as when working against a long lever. Held, or *isometric*, contractions have the effect of increasing blood pressure. In addition, some held positions may cause the performer to hold the breath, dangerously increasing intra-abdominal pressure.

It is generally suggested that full-range movements should be carried out. If the joint is taken through its full range (or through a large proportion of its range) then the muscle will likewise be worked through its full range. This should develop strength, effectiveness and efficiency throughout the whole of the muscle range. In addition, it should also develop or maintain suppleness which will prevent the muscle becoming permanently shortened as can occur in muscles worked regularly within their inner range (see Chapter 2, 'Anatomy, Physiology and Kinesiology Applied to Exercise').

The only exception to this full range recommendation applies to the abdominals. The abdominals should be worked through their inner range purposely to shorten them. Often they become lengthened and weak. Short abdominal muscles are required for holding posture, not just strong muscles.

PROGRESSION AND ADAPTATION RELATING TO EXERCISE INTENSITY

In this context *progression* refers to making an exercise harder. *Adaptation* refers to making an exercise easier.

The Principle of Progression states that we need to make the exercise or training harder if we are to improve our existing fitness and so we have to know how to go about that safely, and what influences intensity and resistance.

On the other hand, it may be that we find a particular exercise too hard (too high an intensity, or too heavy a resistance) and we therefore have to know how to reduce the intensity or resistance. Our body can provide adequate resistance and we have to know how to alter body positions in order to reduce or increase resistance. With most exercises, it is possible to make the exercise harder (progress) or easier (adapt) through a variety of methods.

Progression

Increase repetitions.

Increase range of joint/muscle movement.

Change the body position (with some exercises, changing from a sitting position to a standing position will introduce body weight/gravity as a resistance).

Increase leverage (the resistance arm of the lever can be increased by extending a limb, which will have the effect of increasing the resistance to be overcome by the working muscle).

Adaptation

Decrease repetitions.

Decrease range of joint/muscle movement.

Change body position (possibly to reduce the influence of gravity).

Decrease leverage (the resistance arm of the lever can be shortened by flexing a limb, which will have the effect of reducing the resistance).

8 General Strengthening and Toning Exercises

(Effect, technique, safety and moves to avoid)

Strengthening and toning involves working muscles against resistances. Resistance can be supplied by body weight: different positions can be adopted to provide resistance stress for numerous muscle groups. Body position and limb position can be altered to increase or decrease resistance by employing, reducing or eliminating body weight and gravity, or by increasing or decreasing the leverage.

Some traditional exercises involve body positions and movements which can place excessive and abnormal stress on joints or the spinal column. Whatever the exercise, body position or movement, we have to be careful not to compromise the stability of the spine or place excessive loads on joints by hyperflexion or hyperextension. We should also be certain that the chosen exercise actually works the muscle or muscle group we intend to work.

For those exercising for health-related reasons, correct technique, stability, appropriate intensity, safety and effectiveness are essential.

Sportspersons and athletes with ambitions and championship aspirations may need to train at high intensities, and for strengthening and toning may perform exercises which involve a high element of risk. Their objective is the development of a very high level of fitness *in the short term* in order to achieve their goal. However, such levels of training may jeopardise their *long-term* health and fitness. In the short term a gold medal, championship glory or national selection may be more important than long-term physical well-being.

However, those who reach the top are very few. The majority of athletes simply desire the thrill, enjoyment and satisfaction of their chosen sport. They should consider training methods and exercises which promote long-term well-being and avoid those which may cause progressive physical degeneration. Some exercises, positions and movements need not be performed even by ambitious athletes, as safer and more effective alternatives exist.

In this chapter, and in the following chapters, a variety of exercises are discussed, considering potentially dangerous practice, safer execution and, in most cases, progressions to increase the intensity of resistance.

PRESS-UPS

Starting Position: Crook kneeling, long crook kneeling, or front support.

Effort (positive) phase: Pushing upwards.

Return (negative) phase: Lowering.

Joints moving: Elbow (extension), shoulder (adduction).

Main muscles worked: Triceps (back of upper arm), pectorals (top of chest).

Breathing: Out on the effort, in on the return.

Progressions

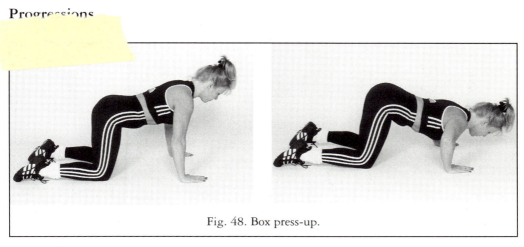

Fig. 48. Box press-up.

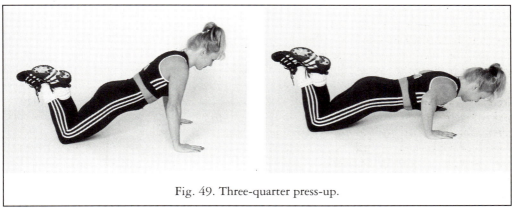

Fig. 49. Three-quarter press-up.

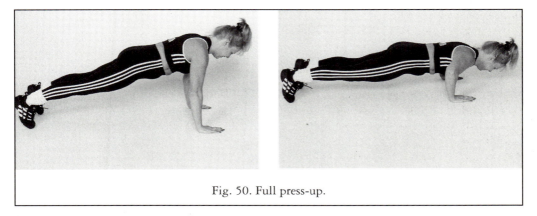

Fig. 50. Full press-up.

Adaptation

Adaptation is needed for those with very limited ability, very little upper body strength, some special needs and in remedial situations.

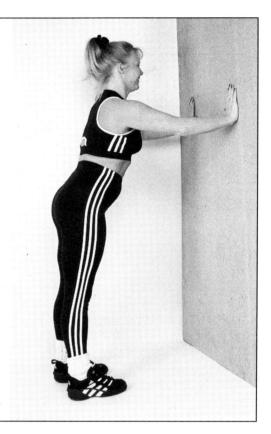

Fig. 51. Press-ups against the wall. The resistance is increased by moving the feet further back from the wall.

Safety and Technique

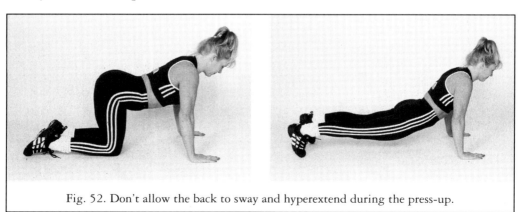

Fig. 52. Don't allow the back to sway and hyperextend during the press-up.

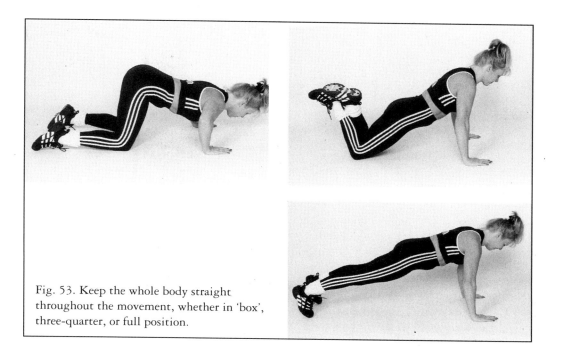

Fig. 53. Keep the whole body straight throughout the movement, whether in 'box', three-quarter, or full position.

Press-up Variations

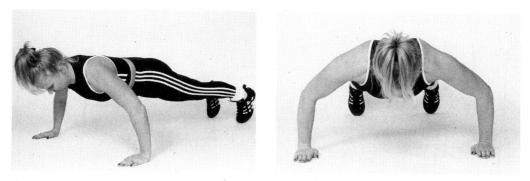

Fig. 54. With the hands placed wide, emphasis is placed on the pectorals.

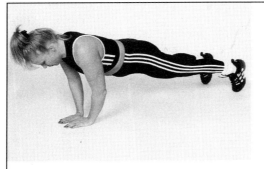

Fig. 55. With the hands placed narrow, emphasis is placed on the triceps.

Fig. 56. With the hands placed further forwards, emphasis is placed on the upper pectorals.

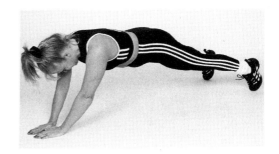

TRICEPS DIPS

Starting position: Crook sitting with hands on the floor behind and elbows bent, fingers towards the body.

Effort phase: Pivot the upper body upwards by straightening the elbows.

Return phase: Bend the elbows slightly to lower the upper body.

Joints moving: Elbows (extension); slight passive movement of hip joint.

Muscles worked: Triceps (back of upper arm).

Breathing: Out on the effort and in on the return.

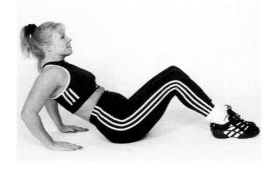

Fig. 57. Triceps dips.

Safety and Technique

Keep the back straight and do not allow to sag on the return.

HIP EXTENSIONS

Start position: Crook kneeling (box position) or crook kneeling but resting on the forearms.

Fig. 58. Hip extension keeping the knee bent: this involves a short lever and minimum resistance.

Effort phase: Lifting the thigh upwards.
Return phase: Lowering the thigh downwards.
Joints moving: Hip joint (extension).
Muscles worked: Hip extensors (gluteals).
Breathing: As occurs naturally and comfortably; suggest out on the effort and in on the return.

Progressions

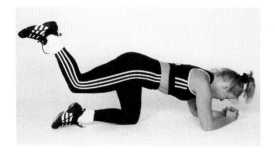

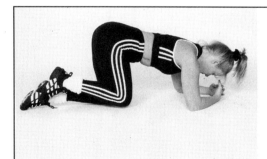

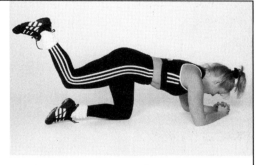

Fig. 59. Hip extension with short lever but covering a greater range of movement.

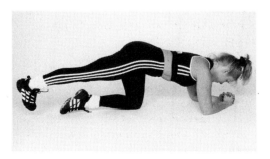

Fig. 60. Hip extension keeping the knee straight. This involves a long lever and more resistance.

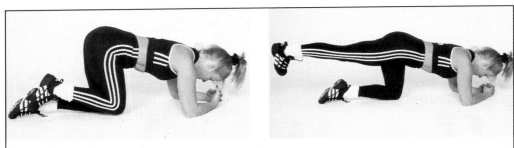

Fig. 61 Hip extension. Knee initially bent but then straightened during lift: covers a greater range and involves a longer lever.

Adaptation

Prone lying, slight hip extension.

Fig. 62. Hip extension in a prone lying position.

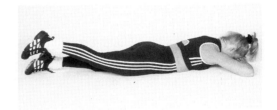

Safety and Technique

Don't kick back vigorously as this builds up momentum which can cause ballistic hyper-extension of the spine and stress the lower back.

Lift the thigh upwards/backwards in a controlled manner, keeping the back flat and straight.

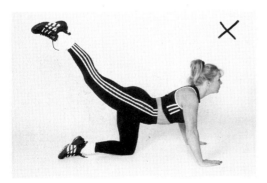

Fig. 63. Vigorous kick-backs are unsafe.

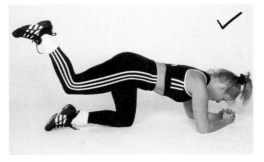

Fig. 64. Controlled lifts backwards are safe.

PELVIC THRUSTS

Start position: Crook lying.

Effort phase: Pushing the pelvis upwards.

Return phase: Lowering the pelvis and back to the floor.

Joints moving: Hips (extension); spinal joints (extension).

Muscles worked: Extensors of the spine; extensors of the hip (gluteals).

Breathing: As occurs naturally and comfortably.

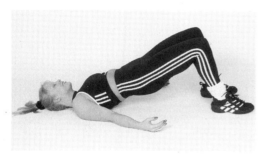

Fig. 65. Pelvic thrusts to exercise the muscles of the back.

Safety and Technique

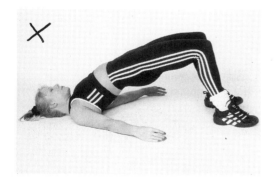

Fig. 66. Don't push up too far into hyper-extension. Keep the movement slow and controlled.

SIDE LEG RAISES (HIP ABDUCTION)

Start Position: Side lying (lower knee comfortably bent, head resting in hand, elbow supporting, other hand on floor in front, weight forwards).

Effort phase: Lifting the thigh upwards and sideways to the body.

Return phase: Lowering the thigh downwards.

Joint moving: Hip joint (abduction).

Muscles worked: Hip abductors (gluteus medius, tensor fascia latae).

Breathing: As occurs naturally and comfortably; suggest out on the effort and in on the return.

Progressions

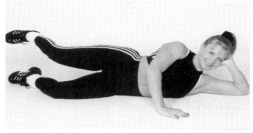

Fig. 67. Side leg raises with the upper knee bent, involving a short lever.

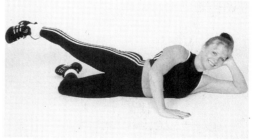

Fig. 68. Side leg raises with the top knee straight, involving a longer lever.

Adaptations

Fig. 69. Upper leg bent, foot on floor, knee lowered and then raised.

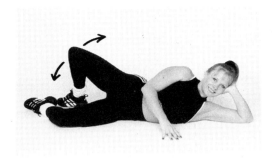

Safety and Technique

Don't allow the body to pike. This reduces the effect as the hip flexors will be worked instead of the hip abductors. Also it can place stress on the lower back.

The correct technique is to push the hips forwards slightly and allow the body weight to roll forwards. Use the arm in front to support. Lift the leg vertically to the side.

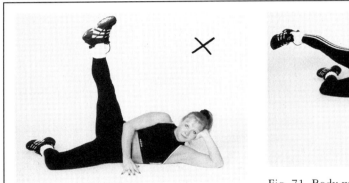

Fig. 70. Piking (not effective).

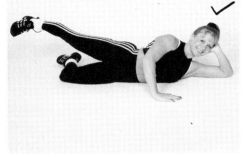

Fig. 71. Body weight and hip slightly forward (correct and effective).

HIP ADDUCTION

Start position: Side lying (as previous exercise).
Effort phase: Lifting the lower leg upwards.
Return phase: Lowering that leg downwards.
Joints moving: Hip joint (adduction).

Muscles worked: Hip adductors (adductor brevis, adductor longus, adductor magnus, gracilis).

Breathing: As occurs naturally and comfortably; suggest out on the effort and in on the return.

Progressions

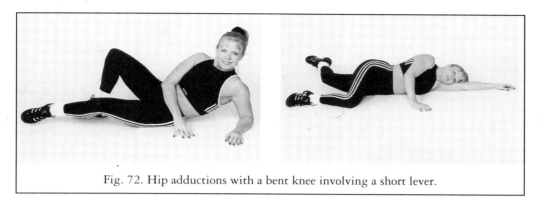

Fig. 72. Hip adductions with a bent knee involving a short lever.

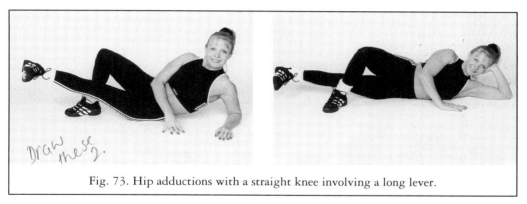

Draw
these 2.

Fig. 73. Hip adductions with a straight knee involving a long lever.

Adaptations

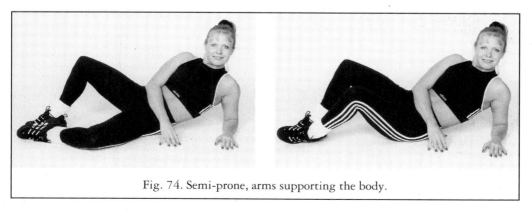

Fig. 74. Semi-prone, arms supporting the body.

Fig. 75. Flat back and bent knee.

In the semi-prone position with the arms supporting the body, one leg has the knee flexed and foot resting on the floor. The other leg is lowered to the floor with the knee flexed. Lift up that leg towards the other leg.

Safety and Technique

Make sure the back is supported and comfortable.

LATERAL THIGH RAISE (ROVER'S REVENGE)

Start position: Prone kneeling.
Effort phase: Lifting the thigh out to the side.
Return phase: Returning the thigh downwards to replace the knee on the floor.
Joint moving: Hip (abduction).
Muscles worked: Hip abductors (gluteus medius; tensor fascia latae).
Breathing: Out on the effort and in on the return.

Progression

Can be performed with a straight leg, but this involves a long lever and is not recommended for beginners.

Safety and Technique

Keep the back flat and straight throughout the movement. It is generally considered that a long lever (straight leg) encourages poor technique and can compromise the safety of the spine.

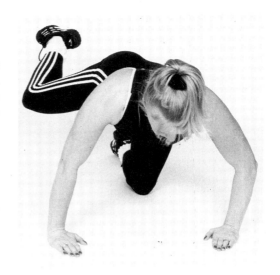

SQUATTING

Starting position: Standing, lower the body weight by bending the knees no more than 90 degrees.
Effort: Lifting the body weight upwards by straightening the knees.
Return: Lowering the body weight down by bending the knees.
Joints moved: Slight dorsiflexion of the ankle joint, knee joint (extension), hip joint (extension).
Muscles worked: Quadriceps, gluteals.

Progression

Only by using additional weights in addition to body weight.

Adaptation

Using a chair; from a sitting position, rise to a standing position and then sit again.

Safety and Technique

Fig. 76. Don't squat too deeply. The knee joint hyperflexes under body weight, placing stress on joint capsule and ligaments.

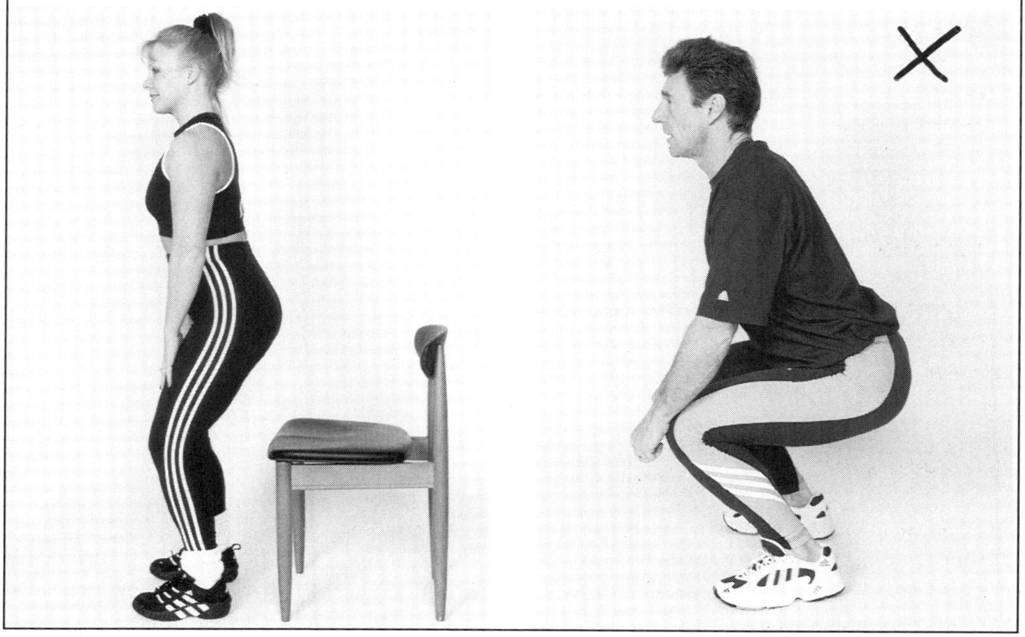

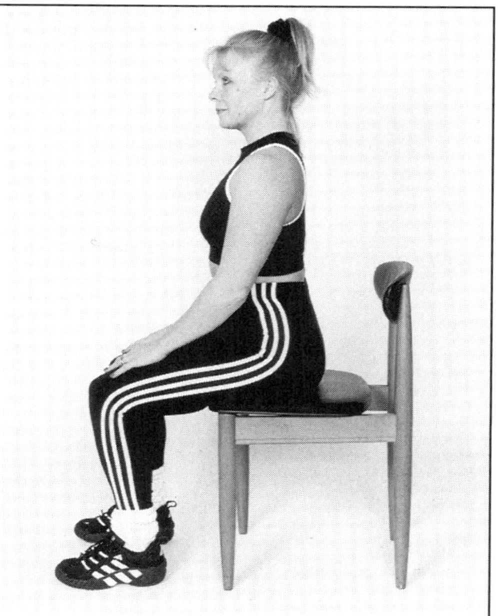

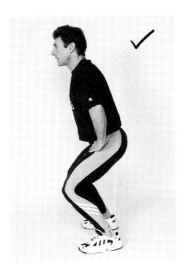

Fig. 77. Squat only to about a 90-degree knee-joint angle.

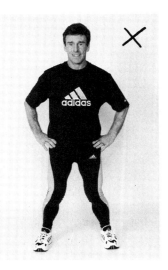

Fig. 78. Don't allow knees to go inwards into a 'knock-kneed' position. This stresses the medial aspect of the knee joint.

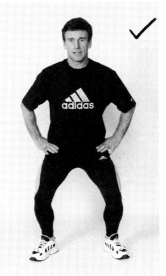

Fig. 79. Keep the knees in line with the toes which should turn outwards slightly.

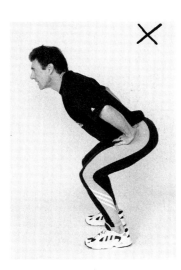

Fig. 80. Don't allow the back to arch and the upper body to lean forwards. This places stress on the lower back.

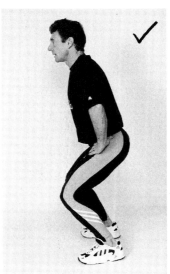

Fig. 81. Keep the back neutral and vertical.

LUNGES

Starting position: Standing; step forwards with one leg into a lunge position.

Effort phase: Push back with the front leg to achieve a standing position.

Return phase: Stepping forwards into the lunge position.

NB. It could be debatable which is the effort phase and which is the return, as this exercise involves both eccentric and concentric muscle work and finishes in a standing position after concentric work. Some people might consider the lunge forward as an effort stage.

Joints moving: (negative) the hip and knee on one side into flexion; (positive) the hip and knee into extension.

Muscles working: Quadriceps and gluteals.

Progression

Only by using additional weights.

Adaptation

See Fig. 82

Safety and Technique

Don't lunge too deeply, allowing the knee to go beyond the line of the end of the toes and therefore hyperflexing the knee joint under weight-bearing load.

Allow only a 90-degree angle at the front knee keeping the knee within the line of the end of the toes.

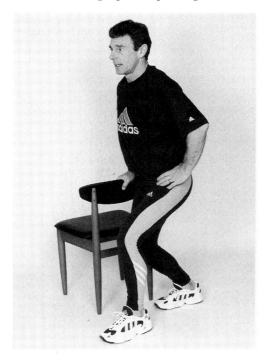

Fig. 82. Split-leg squat using a chair for support.

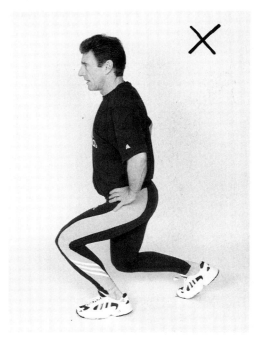

Fig. 83. Deep lunge (unsafe).

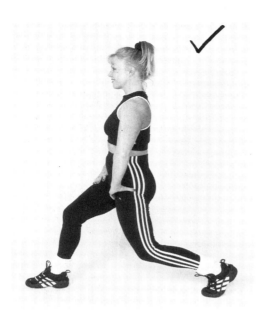

Fig. 84. 90-degree angle lunge (safe).

SIDE BENDS

Starting position: Standing, and then slowly bend to one side from the waist (lateral flexion).

Effort phase: From the side-bending position, straighten up the trunk to the vertical.

Return phase: Lower the trunk down to the side again.

Joints moved: Lumbar spine (lateral flexion).

Muscles worked: Generally the waist region (one side of abdominals, one side of the spinal extensors, quadratus lumborum; there may be some oblique involvement as some of the oblique fibres run vertically, but the main purpose of the obliques is to rotate the trunk).

Progression

Only by holding a dumb-bell weight in one hand and pulling upwards away from the weight.

Adaptation

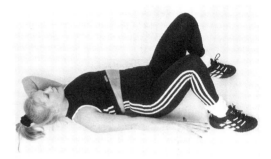

Fig. 85. In a supine crook-lying position, bend to one side and reach with one hand towards the ankle.

Safety and Technique

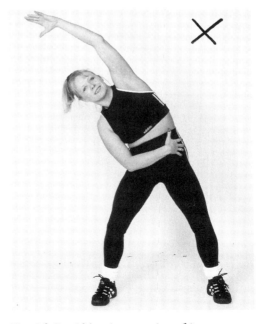

Fig. 86. Rapid leaning over (unsafe).

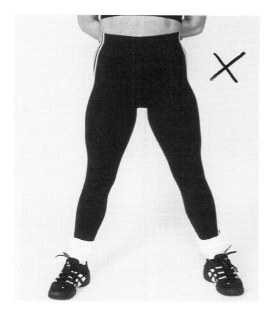 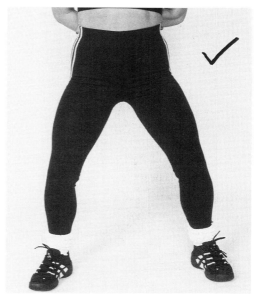

Fig. 87. Don't stand with knees locked and hyperextended. Keep the knees soft throughout the exercise.

Don't lean over to the side quickly with arms above the head. This can create a momentum and reduce control, which can result in ligamemt or muscle strain. The muscles actually try to contract eccentrically because of the stretch reflex.

NB. For abdominal exercises see Chapter 9. For exercises for the back see Chapter 10.

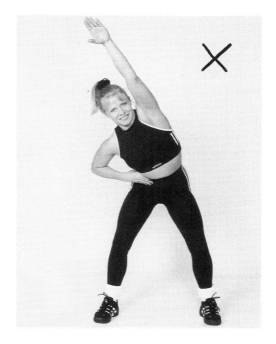

Fig. 88. Don't lean forwards. Keep the back straight throughout the exercise.

9 Abdominal Exercises

(Dangerous practice and safer technique)

SIT-UPS

Sit-ups do not work the abdominals – well, not fully. To exercise a muscle properly we have to work it as a prime mover (that is, the main muscle which contracts to move a joint).

When performing sit-ups, the abdominals are only employed as prime movers for the first 30 degrees of lift from the floor (they flex the spine to curl the trunk). After that the remainder of the movement involves flexion of the hip joint, the legs being fixed and the trunk being lifted up from the hip joint. For this movement, the prime movers are the hip flexor muscles (ilio-psoas), very strong muscles which attach to the lumbar spine at one end, pass through the pelvis, and attach to the inside of the thigh bone (femur) at the other end. As the lumbar spine is not a rigid attachment point but a flexible column, strong tension in the hip flexor muscles can result in tremendous stress on the lumbar spine.

Some people when performing sit-ups do not even return far enough down to work the abdominals through the first 30 degrees of movement, and so no matter how many repetitions are performed the abdominals are not being properly exercised. The return should involve lowering the upper back down to the floor, but the head and shoulders can remain raised slightly to maintain tension in the muscles.

It is true that a person will feel tension in the abdominals as they perform sit-ups, but the muscles are acting as *fixators* (they maintain an isometric contraction to hold the trunk in a flexed position). Prolonged isometric contractions can raise blood pressure which can be dangerous.

A more effective way of exercising the abdominal muscles is to work on the floor *without* the feet anchored, knees bent and feet flat on the floor (this shortens, yet relaxes the hip flexor muscles so that there is no pull on the lumbar spine) and to *curl* the trunk up as far as is possible, keeping the lower back in contact with the floor.

This will develop comparative strength and tone in the abdominals and, if the head and shoulders remain slightly raised on the return, the muscles are worked through their inner range which helps to shorten them. (This is one of the rare cases where we actually work muscles in the inner range so as to shorten them.)

Increases in resistance can be achieved by placing the hands (a) on the thighs so that as the trunk is curled they slide up the thighs to the knees (easy); (b) across the chest (this moves some weight away from the pivot point/fulcrum); (c) by the side of the head/temples (this moves some weight even further from the pivot/fulcrum). Do not place the hands behind the head as there is a tendency to tug which can place strain on the cervical (neck) vertebrae.

If specific strength is required in the abdominals, then an inclined board will cause them to work against gravity and therefore against a greater resistance. In this case the feet will have to be anchored, but the knees *must* be bent to protect the spine. However, a full sit-up need not be performed, but an abdominal curl as described above.

STRAIGHT-LEG RAISES

The hazard of straight-leg raises is that lying on the back and lifting two straight legs is extremely dangerous for the lumbar spine. Once again, the exercise involves hip flexion, the prime mover muscles being the hip flexors and not the abdominals (Mitchell and Dale, 1980; Norris, 1993; Norris, 1994a; Stamford, 1995b). Remember that the hip flexors attach to the flexible lumbar spine.

When we lift two straight legs, the abdominals once again work as fixators (isometric contraction) and the pull of the hip flexors results in an exaggerated forward curve of the lumbar spine (lordosis). Because of the law of levers we must multiply the weight of the resistance arm (the legs) by the length of the lever (or the ratio of the length of the legs to the distance of the hip flexor attachment to the femur below the hip joint, which is the fulcrum). This means that whatever the two legs weigh, we have to multiply that manyfold, and that is the resulting pull/force the hip flexor muscles must exert to lift them. That pull/force is applied to the lumbar spine, which results in a very dangerous situation.

In addition, the effort will usually cause the performer to hold his/her breath, which raises intra-abdominal pressure tremendously and is again very dangerous (Mitchell and Dale, 1980).

To work the abdominals properly in this position (emphasising the lower abdominal fibres), it is not the legs which must be lifted, but the *pelvis*. Either on the flat surface or on an incline, the legs can be tucked towards the chest (this shortens and relaxes the hip flexors) and then the pelvis can be lifted upwards. There is not a great range of movement, but now the abdominal muscles are being worked fully as prime movers.

The abdominal muscles attach to the upper ribs and the pubic crest of the ilium (pelvic bones) and as a result their only action is to flex the spine (curl forwards). They play no part in flexing the hip joint, other than fixing the spine in a rigid position.

Try this: Lie on your back on a flat surface with your legs out straight. You will be able to slide your hands comfortably under the arch in your lower back. This is because the hip flexor muscles are stretched and the resulting tension is pulling at the lumbar spine and causing it to hyperextend (curve forwards). That pull and curve would be greatly increased if you were to lift your two straight legs.

Now bend the legs at the knees with your feet flat on the floor (this has also flexed the hip joint). The upward curve of the lower back has disappeared and you should not be able to slide your hands underneath. The hip flexor muscles are now shortened and comparatively relaxed and there is no pull on the lumbar spine.

THE ROLE OF THE ABDOMINALS

We must consider that the role of the abdominal muscles is not normally to produce movement. Their main purpose is to support the spine and maintain posture in the upper body. They are stabilizers and the oblique abdominals play a major role in stabilization. Therefore abdominal strengthening should include an amount of oblique work, both for internal and external obliques, and for transverse abdominal isolating.

In addition to normal abdominal curls which work the rectus abdominis, we should include some twist curls and abdominal hollowing.

Also, when performing abdominal curls the most effective technique will involve three movements: (i) posterior pelvic tilt, (ii) abdominal hollowing, and (iii) shoulder lift. In this way we will achieve shortening of the abdominal muscles which for posture and a 'flat' stomach is more important than strength (Norris, 1993).

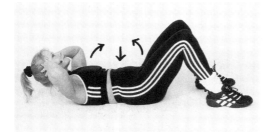

Fig. 89. The three movements of an abdominal curl.

SAFE AND EFFECTIVE ABDOMINAL EXERCISES

Knees are bent and the feet are flat on the floor. Hands may be placed at the side of the head. Lift the head as if looking towards the feet. Curl up by flexing the spine to raise head, shoulders and

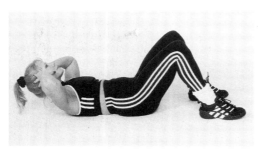

Fig. 90. Abdominal curls (safe and effective).

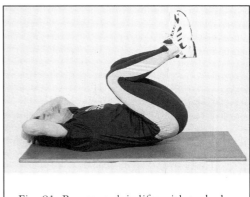

Fig. 91. Reverse pelvic lifts with tucked knees or legs vertical (Safe and effective).

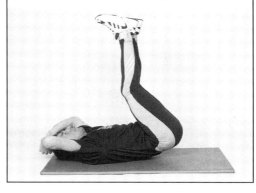

thorax from the floor, but *keep the lower back in contact with the floor.*

Reverse pelvic lifts work the abdominal muscles. Either have the knees tucked or the legs up vertically so as to eliminate the hip flexors. Lift the pelvis. Do not lift so high as to roll onto the back of the neck. Reverse curls emphasize the lower abdominal fibres (Norris, 1993).

Crunches are safe and effective, although slightly more advanced as an amount of skill is required. Lie on the back. Lift the legs and hold them vertically. Place hands by the side of the head and curl up the upper body as with the abdominal curl. Keep lower back in contact with the floor.

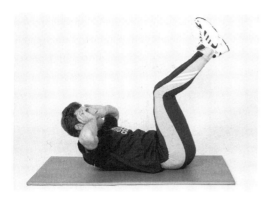

Fig. 92. Crunches (safe and effective).

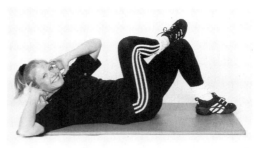

Fig. 94. Twist curls (safe and effective).

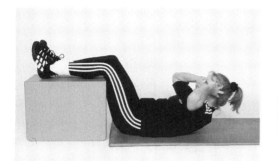

Fig. 93. Crunches with legs up and supported (safe and effective).

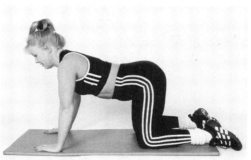

Fig. 95. Abdominal hollowing (kneeling).

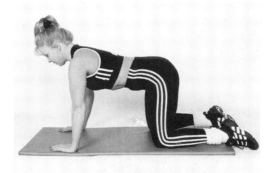

For crunches with legs up and over a bench or on a purpose-built crunch bench there is no need to perform a full sit-up. Keep the lower back in contact with the floor.

Twist curls work the abdominals and the obliques. Lie on the back as for abdominal curls with knees well bent and feet on the floor. The hands are placed by the side of the head at the temples. Lift the right leg and rest the ankle of that leg across the left thigh. This will turn the supported right thigh and knee out slightly. Curl up and rotate the trunk, bringing the left elbow towards the right knee. Keep the right upper arm resting on the floor to take some of the weight and help support the spine. Complete a number of repetitions and repeat for the other side, bringing the right elbow towards the left knee.

Kneel in the 'box' position. Pull up the abdomen by using the deep abdominal muscles (and not by hunching up the spine).

Progressions for Basic Abdominal Exercises

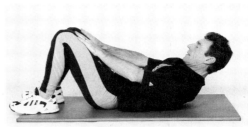

Fig. 97. Abdominal curl with hands on thighs.

thighs, the head and shoulders initially lifted, and the upper body curled, which causes the hands to slide upwards towards the knees. This places some of the body weight towards the fulcrum, therefore producing a comparatively light resistance arm.

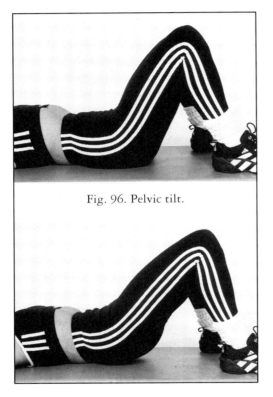

Fig. 96. Pelvic tilt.

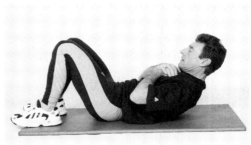

Fig. 98. Abdominal curl with hands across the chest.

The pelvic tilt is one of the easiest methods of abdominal toning and strengthening; it may be particularly suitable in post-natal conditions. Press the lower back down into the floor and tilt the pelvis so that the pubic bone rises. Achieve a slow, steady rhythm when performing repetitions.

The easiest progression for an actual abdominal curl is to have the hands resting on the

Having the hands across the chest is a slightly harder progression because some of the body weight is brought further away from the fulcrum, increasing the weight of the resistance arm.

Hands to the side of the head is a harder progression because the body weight is moved even further away from the fulcrum, increasing the weight of the resistance arm further.

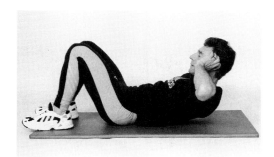

Fig .99. Abdominal curl with hands by the side of the head.

It is important that the hands are placed by the *side* of the head and *not behind the head*. With the hands behind the head there is an instinctive tendency to try to pull, and this may result in strain being placed on the cervical (neck) vertebrae.

NB. For general postural tone it is the shortening of the abdominal muscles that is important, not so much the strengthening (Norris, 1993). It may therefore be sufficient to perform the abdominal curls on a horizontal surface.

Unsafe and Ineffective Abdominal Exercises (not recommended)

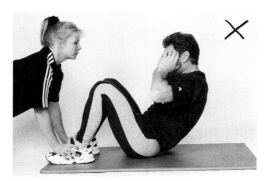

Fig. 100. Full sit-ups (unsafe).

Full sit-ups work the hip flexors as prime movers. The abdominals hold an isometric contraction. This can place stress on the lumbar spine because of the pull of the hip flexors (Champion, 1990).

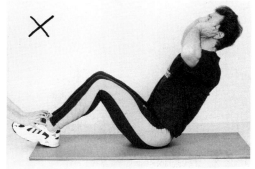

Fig. 101. Full sit-ups with straight back (unsafe and ineffective).

A straight-backed full sit-up pivots from the hip joint, works the hip flexor muscles against a longer lever and stresses the lumbar spine. It does not shorten the abdominals (Norris, 1993).

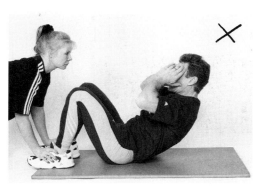

Fig. 102. Sit-ups without returning down far enough (ineffective).

These sit-ups work the hip flexor muscles as prime movers through part of their range causing them to shorten.

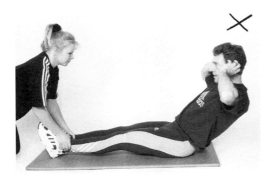

Fig. 103. Straight-leg sit-ups (very dangerous).

Straight-leg sit-ups work the hip flexor muscles from a stretched position against a very long lever and heavy resistance, and therefore place extreme pressure on the lumbar spine.

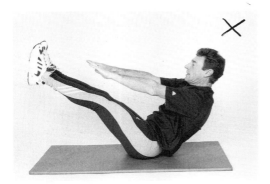

Fig. 104. Piked crunches (dangerous and ineffective).

Piked crunches are performed with straight legs lifted and the upper body lifted so that the lower back rises from the floor, involving high tension in the hip flexors, which places stress on the lumbar spine. They also involve a fast ballistic movement where loss of balance and control can result in traumatic injury (Champion, 1990).

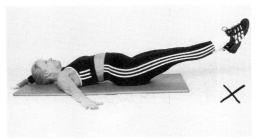

Fig. 105. Straight-leg raises (very dangerous).

Straight-leg raises work the hip flexor muscles against a very long lever and a heavy resistance, and therefore place extreme pressure on the lumbar spine causing hyperextension of the back and 'stretching' of the abdominals. They also cause the performer to hold the breath which develops excessive intra-abdominal pressure and which could be dangerous to some people (Mitchell and Dale, 1980; Champion, 1990; Norris, 1993).

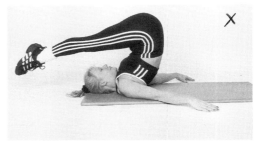

Fig. 106. Straight-leg lifts over the head (very dangerous).

Again, straight-leg lifts work the hip flexor muscles against a very long lever, placing extreme pressure on the lumbar spine initially and, in addition, involve a very dynamic ballistic movement which could damage muscles and intervertebral discs.

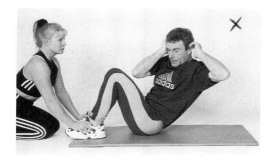

Fig. 107. Full twist sit-ups (dangerous).

Full-twist sit-ups involve rotation of the spine while under flexed tension and pressure from the pull of the hip flexors. It is better to perform twist curls.

Perhaps one of the best recent developments for encouraging correct execution of an abdominal curl and other abdominal exercises is the AB Trainer from Forza. This simple, yet very effective, device consists of a tubular frame which pivots. Lying within the frame the performer has the head resting on a pad and the arms can rest in a variety of positions on the frame including having the elbows on pads if desired. With the knees bent and feet on the floor it allows the ideal movement for an abdominal curl, reverse curl, twist curl and so on, maintains stability of the spine and supports the head for those with weak

neck muscles (Chivers, 1995). A variety of safe positions can be adopted to work both abdominals and obliques.

IMPORTANT TIPS FOR ABDOMINAL EXERCISES

1. Always have bent (flexed) knees when performing abdominal exercises.

2. Perform abdominal exercises in a slow, controlled manner.

3. Breathe out as the trunk is curled up, and breathe in on the return.

4. *Don't hold the breath.*

5. *Don't place the hands behind the head* as the tendency is to tug, thus placing stress on the cervical (neck) vertebrae.

6. If the neck muscles are weak and neck ache is experienced, one hand can be placed behind the head to support the weight.

7. *Don't perform full sit-ups*; abdominal curls are much safer and more effective. It is unnecessary and usually undesirable to raise the trunk more than 30 degrees in abdominal strengthening activities (Howley and Franks, 1992).

8. Keep the head and shoulders slightly raised to maintain tension in the abdominal muscles.

9. Establish what is the purpose of your abdominal training. Developing a flat stomach

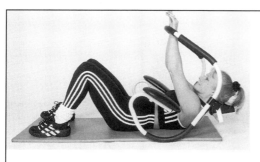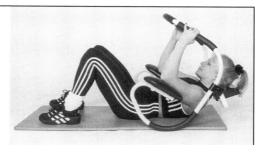

Fig. 108. The AB Trainer from Forza.

and maintaining a properly aligned spine may require *other* muscles to be worked as well, either to be strengthened or to be lengthened.

10. Include exercises for the obliques and the deep abdominal muscles (internal, external and transverse abdominals) such as twist curls and abdominal hollowing.

11. *Don't perform straight leg raises* in an attempt to work the abdominals. This exercise works the hip flexor muscles against a very long lever and therefore a heavy resistance, putting tremendous strain on the lumbar spine and raising intra-abdominal pressure.

12. Emphasize the lower abdominal fibres with reverse curls lifting the pelvis.

13. The main purpose of maintaining good abdominal tone, as well as achieving a flat stomach, is to stabilize and protect the spine. Full sit-up movements will not enhance the function of the spine.

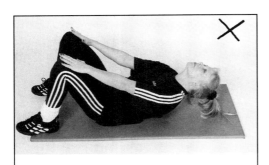

Fig. 109. The head must not drop backwards.

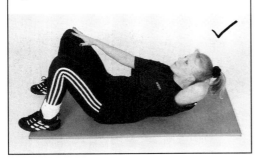

14. *Don't allow the head to drop backwards* during an abdominal curl. Keep the head comfortably forwards/neutral (support the head with one hand if necessary).

ISOMETRIC STABILIZATION

Having previously mentioned the potential dangers of powerful isometric (static/held) contractions, we must remember that the main purpose of the abdominal muscles is to maintain stability and posture. Most of their day-to-day work involves a degree of isometric contraction. The abdominals work primarily to stabilize the pelvis and spine in seated, lying, upright, lifting and moving positions. They are seldom required to lift the upper torso against gravity, yet most people train the abdominals exclusively that way (Cullen, 1997a). It makes sense to include some moderate isometric training for the abdominals as well as isotonic training in our exercise programme.

However, lifting and holding two straight legs is not the answer. Although forcing the abdominals to contract isometrically in an attempt to maintain spinal stability, this exercise is not to be recommended. As previously mentioned, it can place tremendous stress on the lumbar spine and increase pressure dramatically in the abdominal cavity.

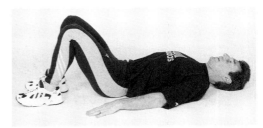

Fig. 110. Starting position with a neutral spine.

Postural stabilizing (or functional abdominal) exercises should be performed along with isotonic abdominal curls and twist curls. Attention should be given to correct breathing and the development of the transverse abdominals, which are respiratory muscles and also maintain the position of the internal organs.

In the basic starting position, lying supine with the knees bent and feet flat on the floor, the arms comfortably by the side, try to find a position of the spine which is considered neutral. This will be somewhere between hyperextension (arched lumbar spine) and the lower back pressed down into the floor. The lower back will probably be only lightly touching the floor.

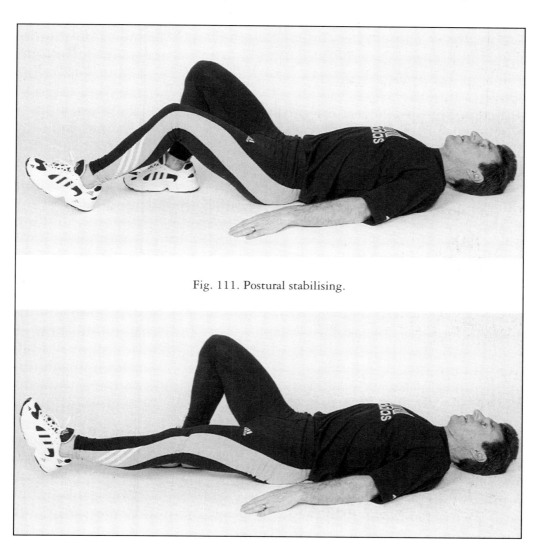

Fig. 111. Postural stabilising.

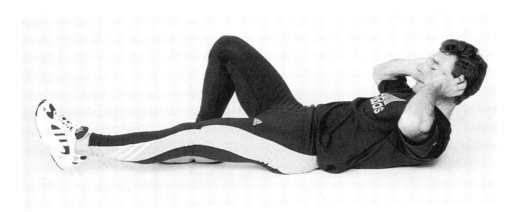

Fig. 112. Postural stabilising, progression.

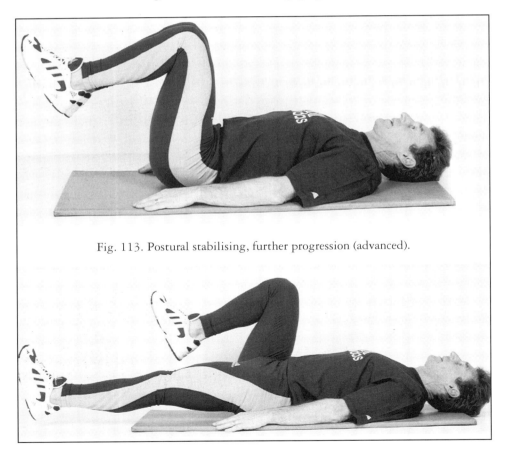

Fig. 113. Postural stabilising, further progression (advanced).

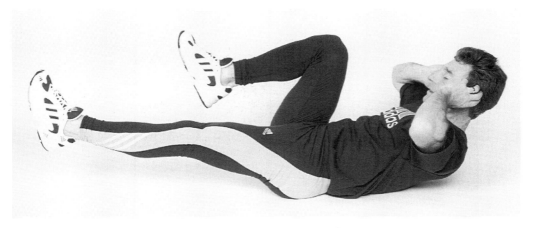

Fig. 114. Postural stabilising, a very advanced progression.

While inhaling, the chest and stomach should rise; while exhaling, the chest and stomach should fall and the abdomen is pulled in, involving contraction of the transverse abdominals. Throughout, a neutral spine should be maintained.

Having mastered this simple technique of correct breathing, a number of postural stabilizing (functional) exercises can be performed.

Exhale and pull in the stomach while sliding one leg out, maintaining a neutral spine. Inhale as the leg is returned and then repeat with the other leg (Fig. 111).

The next progression is to perform an abdominal curl at the same time as the leg slides out and the stomach is compressed. Exhale as the leg slides out and the torso is lifted. Inhale on the return (Fig. 112).

A further progression is to have the legs raised and bent. With the knees in line with the hips, this eliminates the hip flexors and reduces pull on the lumbar spine. The arms are placed by the

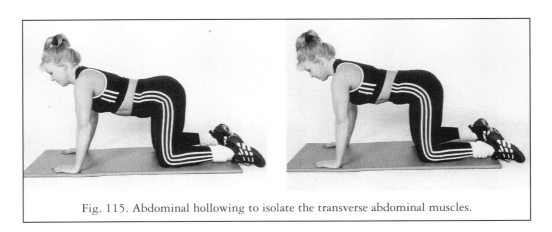

Fig. 115. Abdominal hollowing to isolate the transverse abdominal muscles.

side of the body and the spine is in a neutral position. Exhale while compressing the abdomen and slide one leg out. Inhale on the return and repeat with the other leg (Fig. 113).

A further progression is to add an abdominal curl to the above-mentioned exercise. Curl the torso as the leg slides out. Inhale on the return and repeat with the other leg. (Cullen, 1997b).

Although working the abdominals generally in a more functional capacity, the above exercises do not isolate the main abdominal stabilizers, the transverse abdominals. Developing effective functional stability will require exercising to isolate the transverse abdominals in addition to performing trunk curls and twist curls. The exercise to achieve this involves abdominal hollowing.

In a prone-kneeling position, pull the tummy upwards by contracting the abdominal muscles. This is held for a few seconds, then relax and repeat (Fig. 115).

Do not bend the back. Keep the spine parallel to the floor throughout and pull up the tummy. Instinct may cause you to breathe out during the initial contraction. This is natural because the transverse abdominals do assist with forced expiration. However, do not then hold the breath. Try to breathe normally throughout the exercise and when holding the contraction.

As you become more proficient at abdominal hollowing, you will be able to perform this exercise at any time, even in a standing or sitting position.

10 Exercises for the Back

As with all muscle groups it is important to maintain a balance in strength and tone between antagonistic pairs or opposing muscles. The muscles which oppose the abdominals (rectus abdomini) are the spinal extensors (erector spinae).

However, we must be very cautious with exercises for the back and consider the role of the spinal muscles. As with the abdominals, their main role is one of stabilization. All the muscles of the trunk work to support the spine through its ranges of movement and in a variety of held positions. Ideally, they should support the spine in its neutral position and maintain its correct natural curves. Over-enthusiasm for exercising the deep extensor muscles of the back can result in over-shortening of those muscles, exaggerated curves of the spine and poor posture – as can neglect of those muscles.

The side and back views of the spine show how

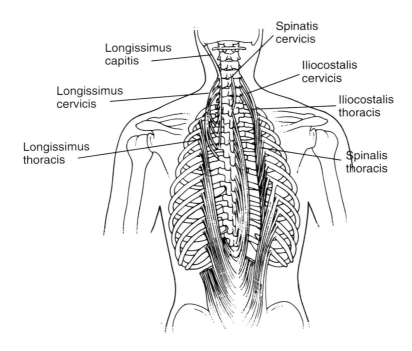

Fig. 116. The extensor muscles of the spine (collectively erector spinae).

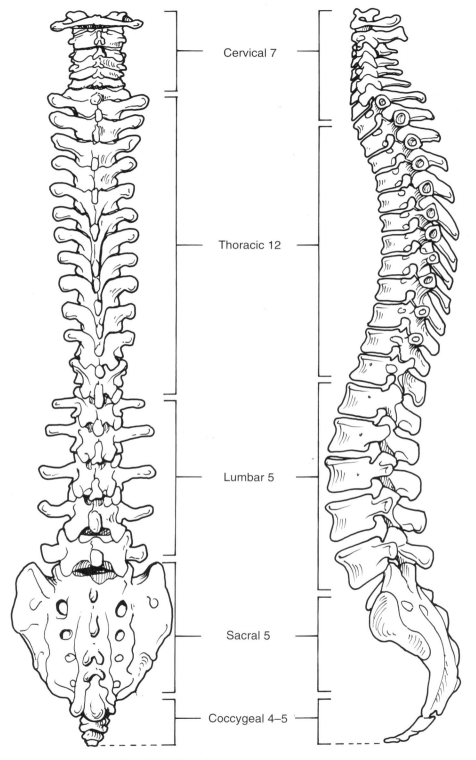

Cervical 7

Thoracic 12

Lumbar 5

Sacral 5

Coccygeal 4–5

Fig. 117. The spine and its natural curves.

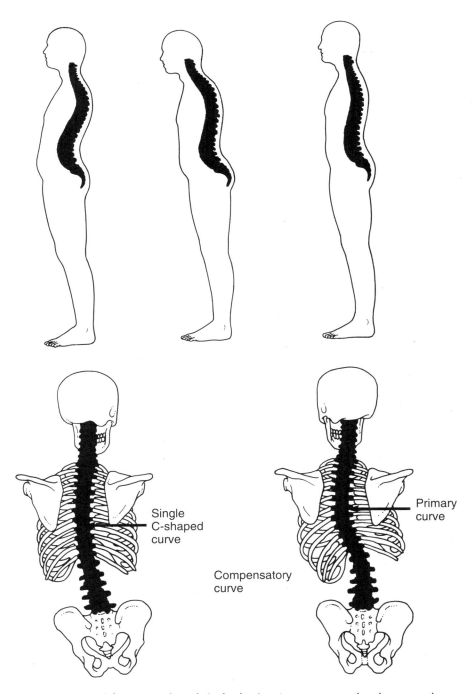

Single
C-shaped
curve

Primary
curve

Compensatory
curve

Fig. 118. The spine viewed from the side and the back, showing exaggerated and unnatural curves.

the normal curves can be exaggerated and how lateral flexion can develop through habitual poor posture, repetitive occupational posture, and/or incorrect or inappropriate exercise.

Hyperextensions are generally not recommended to be done on a regular, repetitive basis and definitely not in a ballistic fashion. Conservative practice of the following spinal extensions may be indicated, although a person's existing posture should be examined and in some cases those the spinal extensor muscles may actually need lengthening.

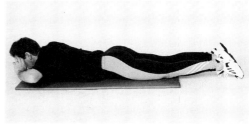

Fig. 120. Place arms by side of body, hands towards feet, or rest hands on buttocks.

TRUNK RAISES

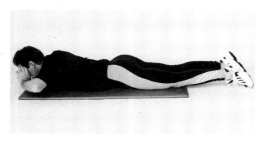

Fig. 119. Trunk raises.

In a trunk raise, lying face down, the upper body is lifted up from the floor in a slow, controlled manner without jerking and without forcing too high. Keep the stomach and lower ribs in contact with the floor. Lift the upper chest and shoulders only a couple of inches (approximately 5cm) to a count of two, hold for a count of one and then return. Do not lift the head backwards, hyperextending the neck. *Keep the legs and feet on the floor.*

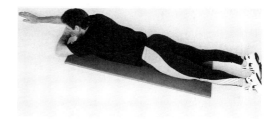

Fig. 121. Place hands by side of head or under chin with fingers interlocked.

Fig. 122. Stretch one arm out forward in front of head.

Progressions

Three progressions increase the difficulty level or resistance by increasing the leverage:

For health-related fitness it may not be necessary to perform trunk raises beyond progression 2 with the hands under the chin.

Tips for Trunk Raises

1. Perform trunk raises in a slow, controlled manner.

2. *Don't* perform full trunk hyperextensions by lifting both trunk and legs together.

3. Lift only the upper chest and shoulders, and only about two inches/5cm.

4. *Don't* pull the head backwards, hyperextending the neck.

5. Choose the amount of resistance/leverage (position of the arms/hands) that suits your requirements and do not strain.

PELVIC THRUSTS

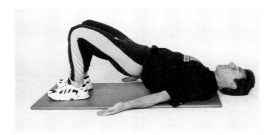

Fig. 123. Pelvic thrust.

From a crook-lying position, push the pelvis upwards by contracting the gluteals and the spinal extensors. *Do not* push up too far into extreme hyperextension. The movement involves hip and back extension, although the muscles being worked are facing downwards.

SAFE SPINAL STABILIZATION

Another method for strengthening the back involves lying prone (face down) on a bench with the hips at the end of the bench. The feet are anchored by a partner or other securing device. The weight of the upper body is supported on the arms with the hands resting on the floor. Take the hands away and hold the upper body horizontal for a few seconds (*do not* lift up into hyperextension) and then return the hands to the floor to take the weight again. This works the spinal extensors as stabilisers by holding an isometric contraction. As isometric contractions increase blood pressure during the hold, do not hold for too long.

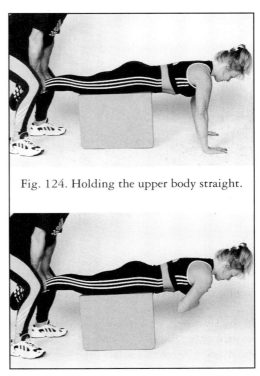

Fig. 124. Holding the upper body straight.

UNSAFE EXERCISES

One exercise *not recommended* is a full trunk hyperextension where both the trunk and legs are lifted off the floor simultaneously and often performed vigorously. The upper body and the lower body form two long levers with the lower back as the fulcrum. The muscle contraction required to lift both of these simultaneously is enormous and can cause injury to the lower back (Egger *et al.*, 1988). Repetition of this exercise on a regular basis may cause micro-trauma to the intervertebral discs and the possibility of nerve impingement. Such injuries or conditions do not usually occur suddenly, but manifest over a long period of time and may cause pain and suffering in the future. However, acute inflammation of the facet joints can occur along with chronic degeneration. In addition, over-shortening of the spinal muscles may occur, which increases lumbar lordosis and develops poor posture.

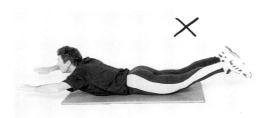

Fig. 125. Full Trunk Hyperextensions (dangerous and not recommended).

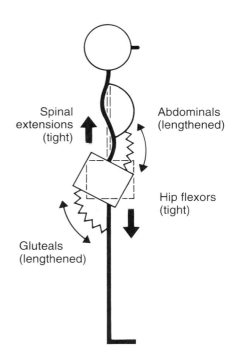

Spinal extensions (tight)

Abdominals (lengthened)

Hip flexors (tight)

Gluteals (lengthened)

Fig. 126 Exaggerated lumbar lordosis: tilted pelvis because of shortened spinal extensors and hip flexors and lengthened abdominals and gluteals.

Although discussed under the heading of 'abdominal exercises', another exercise not recommended because of the danger it presents to the lumbar spine is straight-leg lifts while lying on the back. The forced hyperextension of the lumbar spine with this exercise dramatically increases the stress on the facet joints of the spine (Norris, 1993).

In some cases the lower spinal extensors may have over-shortened together with the hip flexors. The top of the pelvis is tilted forwards and the lordotic curve in the lower back exaggerated. This will require shortening of the abdominals and gluteals and stretching of the spinal extensors and hip flexors (Lycholat, 1995a).

An exaggerated curve in the upper back (kyphosis) will result from shortened pectorals and lengthened extensor muscles of the back, including rhomboids between the shoulder blades (scapulae). The pectorals will require stretching and the opposing muscles at the back will require strengthening. It is important, though, that a person with an exaggerated kyphotic curve should be checked by a doctor for degenerative bone disease (Baird, 1996).

Once again, this illustrates the need for a balanced exercise programme. Through a balanced programme, an appropriate stretching programme and the adoption of good posture techniques you will endeavour to stave off injuries and maximize the efficiency of your training (Baird, 1996).

The lower back is one of the most injury-prone areas of the body. Correct technique and posture when performing exercises for the back can help reduce the problem of lower back pain (Champion, 1990).

Throw Away the Broom Handle:

Visit a typical modern health club, state of the art, clean, attractive, with the most up-to-date resistance and aerobic equipment but, in the corner, leaning against the wall and looking most out-of-place in its sophisticated surroundings, is a wooden broom handle! Why? Well, some members have a desire to place it across their shoulders and, with arms stretched along it, twist the body vigorously from side to side. They are obviously under the impression that this traditionally practised exercise is of some benefit, perhaps to the waist or back.

In fact, it should be included in the list of controversial exercises which may do more harm than good. It may even be considered contra-indicated, for although the human trunk is designed to rotate significantly, it was not designed for high repetitions of the end-of-range ballistic twists that occur with this exercise.

The broom handle, or any other bar placed across the shoulders, or outstretched arms, produces a turning force and torque about the axis of rotation (the spine). The inertia developed results in a vigorous ballistic twisting movement which may cause muscle fibre damage to the obliques, but is more likely to produce tugging, stretching and tearing of the many tiny spinal ligaments. In addition, the rapid and extreme rotation of the spine with the

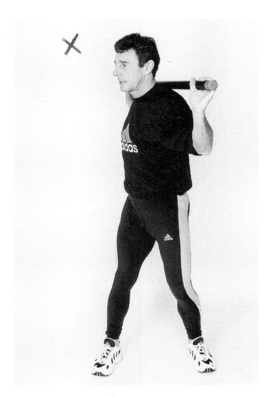

Fig. 127. Trunk rotations with a bar across the shoulders (dangerous).

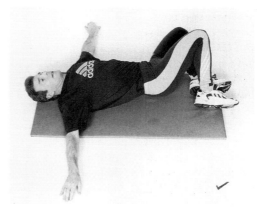

Fig. 128. Lower body rotations in a crook-lying position for mobilising the spine (safer).

89

upper body weight pressing down produces a sheering force in the intervertebral discs. Imagine holding a piece of sponge with one hand on the top and one hand on the bottom and then twisting it.

If mobilizing the spine is the objective, then a far safer exercise involves trunk rotations in a supine position; lying on your back, knees bent and feet flat on the floor, arms out to the side like a crucifix. The lower body is rotated in a controlled manner so that the knees go down to the floor on one side and then the other.

In a horizontal position there is no compressive force down through the spine and intervertebral discs. If performed comparatively slowly and under control, the sheering force is reduced.

This exercise is often prescribed by physiotherapists to increase mobility of the spine and to alleviate lower back pain. The broom handle method may actually be the cause of acute back pain because of creeping or progressive microtrauma and the development of arthritis.

In the gymnasium, the most useful exercise we can perform with the broom handle would be to attach a mop head to the end of it and clean the changing-room floor. Then put it back in the broom cupboard where it belongs.

Part Three: Stretching

11 The Theory and Scientific Background to Stretching

We stretch to develop flexibility and suppleness and to improve the efficiency of the muscles to lengthen and to handle eccentric contraction (lengthening under resistance).

Flexibility may be defined as the range of movement at joints, and stretching increases the range of movement at joints (Smith, 1994).

Suppleness may be defined as the lengthening ability of the muscles, which will contribute towards increased flexibility at the joints (Smith, 1994).

The sports person or athlete needs to develop suppleness and flexibility to (a) enhance performance, and (b) to reduce the likelihood of injury. In health-related fitness a better range of movement makes everyday tasks easier and reduces the risk of injury from everyday stresses. Stretching trains the muscles to relax, increases their elongation potential, and therefore increases range of movement at joints.

It is ironic, but muscles which cause movement can also restrict movement because of negative tension. This is why we include stretching exercises in our fitness programme to relieve that tension in the muscles. Relaxed muscles, or muscles that can lengthen efficiently, allow a better range of movement at the joints. Moderate static stretching may be useful to relieve neuromuscular tension (A.C.S.M., 1986).

We may experience nervous tension and then muscles will tighten up. Driving in heavy traffic, being late for work or appointments, difficult situations at work or at home, problems, traumas, crises, decision-making and so on can all contribute to making us feel tense, nervous and tired.

Negative muscle tension expends wasted energy. Skeletal muscle will be affected and we feel pain and aching from fatigued muscles. The will to move and the ability to move diminish.

Our muscles are in a state of contraction for most of the time. They work by contracting.

They may often be required to work repeatedly within their inner range and thus become shortened (they lose their ability to lengthen fully). This will have an adverse effect on eccentric contraction.

By stretching muscles we allow them to relax to their full length so that the full range of the muscle is employed instead of it remaining in a semi-contracted, tight, mid-range state. Physical benefits should become obvious in that we will be able to move better, feel physically more relaxed and be more able to cope with physical tasks. In addition, getting the muscles to relax can have psychological benefits too by possibly easing state of mind, increasing confidence and the ability to cope with mental tasks.

Muscles have elastic properties in that they have the ability to alter their length and return. They are not like rubber elastic which stretches out and then relaxes back to its original shortened state. Muscles are contractile; they are relaxed when at length and work by contracting.

When we stretch a muscle it is not quite the same as stretching rubber elastic. We actually open the muscle out to its full length and then take it a bit further. This does create a tension in the muscle for a few moments, but a different tension than when it contracts. Muscles spend a lot of time in a contracted state and need to be opened out and stretched regularly.

Stretching should always be carried out before any form of physical activity – whether it be an exercise class, training session, or competitive sport. Stretching should form a vital part of the warm-up, but it is important to include the stretching *after* the muscles are well warmed up (Norris, 1994b; Smith, 1994). The degree of stretch should not be so extreme as to cause significant pain (A.C.S.M., 1986).

If muscle fibres are going to tear they will usually tear on sudden lengthening or powerful eccentric contraction. With a forceful, explosive movement, the antagonist muscle, which is lengthening to control the movement, may not be able to cope with the speed and force and fibres may be torn. Regular stretching of muscles enables them to cope more efficiently with this quick and powerful lengthening that can occur in exercise and sporting situations.

TYPES OF STRETCHING

Basically there are two types of stretching:

1. Ballistic Stretching

This includes mobilizing exercises and ballistic bounces.

(a) Mobilizing exercises which consist of gentle joint movements to stimulate the secretion of synovial fluid and to warm the muscles affecting that joint.

(b) Ballistic bounces involve a muscle being opened to its full length and then stretched by bouncing movements. This method of stretching is *not* recommended as it can cause damage to the connective tissue in the muscle, may invoke a stretch reflex, and may cause damage to muscle fibres.

2. Static Stretching

During static stretching we open the muscle to its full length and gently stretch it a little further, holding the position for a length of time. Static stretching can be further sub-divided into active and passive stretching.

(a) *Active stretching* is when the performer carries out the stretch and holds the position.

(b) *Passive stretching* is when the limb is moved and the stretch position is held by another person. Some authorities consider that passive stretching also includes exercises where gravity or any outside force causes a muscle to be stretched rather than the concentric contraction of an opposing muscle (Alter, 1990; Smith, 1994).

With passive stretching we can carry out PNF stretching (Propreoceptive Neuromuscular Facilitation), sometimes referred to as contract-relax stretching because, having held a muscle in a stretch position for a length of time, we then get the muscle to contract forcefully and isometrically against a strong resistance for a few seconds and then get it to relax and lengthen further. This phenomenon occurs because we invoke an *inverse stretch reflex* (a neurological response) in the muscle which causes the muscle fibres to relax in response to high tension.

PNF stretching is perhaps better carried out passively with the assistance of another person although it can be performed actively. Either way, the muscle to be stretched is moved slowly into its maximum (yet comfortable) lengthened position and is held there for a number of seconds. Then the muscle is contracted isometrically for about five seconds against a resistance from the partner. The tension developed is sensed by the golgi tendon organ (GTO, a propreoceptor in the musculo-tendon junction) which excites the inverse stretch reflex and gets the muscle fibres to relax. When the isometric contraction (and therefore the tension) is stopped, the muscle will lengthen further because of the relaxing effect of the inverse stretch reflex.

There are two methods of PNF stretching: *contract relax* (CR) and *contract relax agonist contract* (CRAC). With the CR PNF method the partner initially assists with the stretch, then provides the resistance, and then assists with the second stretch which should go much further if a good response has been achieved from the GTO and inverse stretch reflex.

With the CRAC method the same procedure is carried out but after the isometric contraction the performer uses the opposing muscle as a prime mover (agonist) to pull the muscle to be stretched into a further stretch. Therefore this part of the stretch is performed actively.

Stretch Reflex

Within muscles are proprioceptors in the form of muscle spindles. Muscle spindles resemble a coiled wire around muscle fibres. When a muscle is stretched (even the minutest lengthening) the stretch is sensed by the spindle and a message is sent via a sensory nerve to the central nervous system. A message returns via a motor nerve to the muscle fibre telling it to contract. Stretch reflex is therefore the basis of muscle tone.

Inverse Stretch Reflex

If a muscle is subjected to excessive tension, as might happen when suddenly exposed to a very heavy resistance, the excessive tension is sensed by other proprioceptors, this time in the muscle–tendon junction. These sensory organs are known as golgi tendon organs (GTO). When the GTO senses excessive tension a message is sent to the central nervous system and a message returns telling the muscle fibres to relax. In this way, it acts as a safety device, protecting the muscle fibres from forces that could otherwise damage them.

Reciprocal Inhibition (reciprocal relaxation)

When a muscle contracts, its opposing muscle relaxes. If there is tension in a muscle, it can be relaxed by holding a contraction in its opposing muscle (Mitchell, 1987). This is a reflex and will occur when employing the CRAC method of PNF stretching (Lycholat, 1995b).

STRETCHING FOR DEVELOPMENT OR MAINTENANCE

We can stretch muscles to *develop flexibility* or to *maintain existing flexibility.*

When we stretch muscles we are attempting to maintain or increase the lengthening ability of the muscle. In order to increase the ability of the muscle to lengthen we need to stretch the connective tissue within the muscle and increase the elongation potential of the muscle fibres.

The bulk of the muscle consists of bundles of muscle fibres bound together by an inelastic connective tissue made mainly of collagen.

Ballistic stretching does not increase the length of the connective collagen tissue, though it does have an effect on the muscle fibres. By bouncing a muscle therefore, we can actually cause damage to the collagen fibres which can result in muscle pain and not necessarily any increase in the relaxation potential of the belly of the muscle. Bouncing can cause more stretch than your tissues can handle. This can lead to small tears in muscles and connective tissue. The tears heal by scarring, which shortens the muscle and limits flexibility (Pullig-Schatz, 1994).

Ballistic stretching may be indicated for certain sports and activities. In karate, dance and gymnastics for example, high-velocity movements are involved and have to be practised. Participants of such activities may regularly perform some ballistic stretching, and habituation causes an increase in the threshold level at which the stretch reflex occurs. However, such regular ballistic stretching should be built up on a base of static stretching.

Although the collagen fibre is comparatively inelastic, when warm it can become more pliable and can be permanently elongated. If cold it is brittle and can be damaged, and this is the reason why stretching exercises should always be carried out in warm conditions and when the muscle is well warmed up. If stretches are being carried out as part of the preparatory warm-up before training or sport they should be performed *after* the mobilizing and pulse raiser components of the warm-up (Norris, 1994b; Smith, 1994).

Maintenance stretches might be those stretches carried out as part of the warm-up before activity, or as part of the cool-down at the end of the activity.

This type of stretching will involve slowly opening the muscle to its full length, stretching it gently a bit further so that an amount of comfortable tension is developed and holding the stretch position for between 7 to 10 seconds.

If stretching for the development of flexibility we need to hold the stretch much longer – at least 20 to 30 seconds, and perhaps 30 to 60 seconds (Smith, 1994; Lycholat, 1995b). This can be carried out in three progressive stages (the progressive stretch method):

1. Very slowly and gently ease the muscle into a comfortable lengthened position. This allows the muscle to become desensitized (it cancels out the stretch reflex) and become accustomed to the lengthened state. Hold this comfortable stretch for about 7 seconds.

2. Then maintain the position but slightly increase the stretch tension very slowly and gently and hold for another 7 seconds. This now allows the warm collagen connective tissue fibres to stretch (known as 'creeping').

3. Maintain the stretch position but now increase the stretch tension slightly more and hold for a further 7 seconds. This allows the muscle fibres to elongate along with the connective tissue. In this way you will have held

the stretch position for approximately 21 seconds.

Anderson (1989) discussed starting with an 'easy stretch' where you feel *mild tension* and relax as the stretch is held for 10 to 30 seconds. Then move a fraction until you again feel mild tension and hold for 10 to 30 seconds. Any tension should diminish; if not, ease off slightly.

Not all muscles of the body require developmental stretching, but those major muscles prone to shortening, and which will therefore restrict full range of movement in the joints they affect, should be stretched.

Hamstrings at the back of the thigh, calf muscles at the back of the lower leg and adductors of the inner thigh may be in need of developmental stretching. Most sports and activities involving a high percentage of leg power will require the athlete to develop suppleness in quadriceps (front of the thigh), hamstrings (back of the thigh), calf muscles – gastrocnemius and soleus (back of the lower leg), anterior tibial muscles (front of the lower leg), gluteals (buttocks), adductors (inner thigh), and

hip flexors – ilio-psoas (deep muscles attached to the lumbar spine and to the inside of the femur; they lift up the thigh, and the stretch tension will be felt in the groin/top thigh region).

All the above muscles should be stretched as part of the warm-up (after gentle, low-intensity activity to warm the muscles), and again at the end of a training session or competition as a vital part of the cool-down. Stretching thus becomes an important part of the training programme.

GOLDEN RULES FOR STRETCHING CORRECTLY

1. Stretch *warm* muscles.

2. *Do not bounce.*

3. Ease the muscle slowly into a comfortable stretch position and hold for a few seconds.

4. Then slightly increase the stretch tension and hold for a few seconds more.

5. *Do not overstretch:* keep within the limits of pain.

12 Stretching Exercises

FOR THE LOWER BODY

The Calf Muscles at the Back of the Lower Leg (gastrocnemius and soleus)

If we stretch the calf with the knee extended we emphasise gastrocnemius; if we stretch the calf with the knee flexed we emphasise soleus.

For stretching the calf, stand with one foot forward and one foot back, both feet pointing forwards (it is important that the back foot is

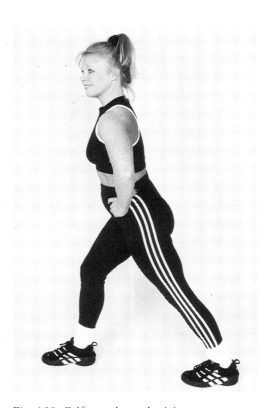

Fig. 129. Calf stretch emphasizing gastrocnemius.

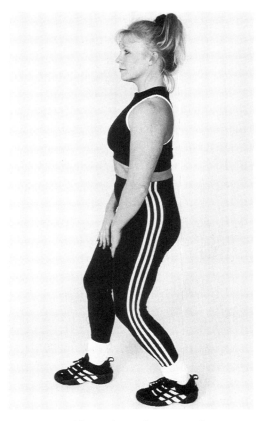

Fig. 130. Calf stretch emphasizing soleus.

pointing directly forwards). Bend the knee of the front leg and allow your body weight to come forward over that leg. Keep the back leg straight and the heel down to the floor. Hold that position for about 7 to 10 seconds and the stretch will occur in the calf region of the back leg, emphasizing the gastrocnemeus muscle. Change over legs and repeat.

This free-standing calf stretch is a gentle stretch and is often performed as part of the pre-stretch and post-stretch components of an exercise to music session.

From the previously mentioned position, bend the back leg slightly and bring the body-weight backwards so that it is over the back leg (often the position is described as sitting on an imaginary bar stool). Keep the heel of the back foot down on the floor, hold for about 7 to 10 seconds, and the stretch is now emphasized in the soleus muscle of the calf.

Again, the above-mentioned free-standing calf stretch for soleus is often used as part of the pre-stretch and post-stretch components of an exercise to music session.

Stand facing a wall with the feet together about one metre away from the wall. Lean towards the wall supporting the body weight with the outstretched arms. Allow the heels to lower down to the floor. This is a comfortable stretch emphasizing gastrocnemius (the outer of the calf muscles).

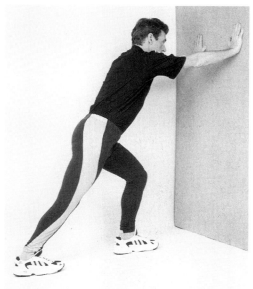

Fig. 132. Calf stretch, against wall (2).

Stand facing a wall with both feet about one metre away from the wall. Place one foot forward closer to the wall. As with the previous exercise, allow the heel of the rear foot to lower towards the floor and hold for about 7 to 10 seconds, thus stretching the gastrocnemius muscle of that rear leg. As flexibility increases

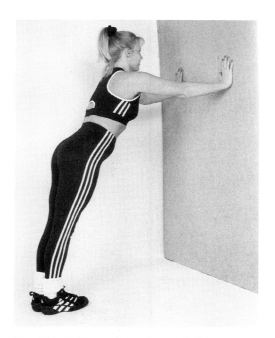

Fig. 131. Calf stretch, against wall (1).

you can move the rear foot further back to increase the stretch, as well as bending the arms to lower the body towards the wall. Change over legs and repeat.

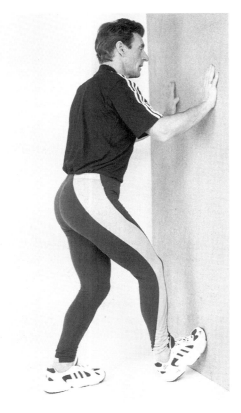

Fig. 133. Calf stretch, against wall (3).

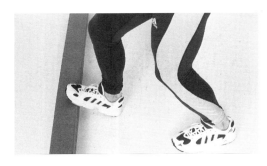

Stand facing a wall, but this time a little closer to the wall. Place one foot up to the wall with the foot dorsi-flexed (toes up) against the wall and the heel on the floor. Flex the knee of that leg so that it moves towards the wall and the stretch will be felt in the lower part of the calf muscles of that leg (soleus is emphasized). Hold for about 7 to 10 seconds. Change over legs and repeat.

The above stretch (emphasizing soleus) can also be performed by placing a foot against a curb so that the toes are on the top of the curb, and then bending the knee of that leg.

Both gastrocnemius and soleus (the calf muscles) insert to the heel bone (calcaneus) via one common tendon – the Achilles tendon, but they have separate attachment points at their origin at the top of the muscle.

Because gastrocnemius attaches by two heads to the femur *above* the knee joint, it is emphasized when stretched with the knee extended (straight).

Soleus attaches to the back of the tibia (the shin bone) *below* the knee joint and is emphasized when stretched with the knee flexed (bent).

Anterior Tibial Muscle at the Front of the Lower Leg

Kneel on the floor with the toes pointing back so that you are sitting on your heels. Allow your body weight to press downwards to exaggerate the plantar-flexion of the feet.

Body weight can be adjusted to reduce or increase the stretch tension. Remember, keep within the limits of pain and adjust body weight by lifting slightly off the heels to start with.

The anterior tibial muscle can also be stretched while stretching the quadriceps muscles in a standing or prone (face down) lying position, as will be evident in the next section.

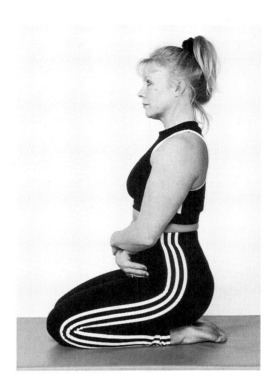

Fig. 134. Anterior tibial stretch.

and gently pull that foot towards the buttock. Press the hip down towards the floor. Hold the position for about 7 to 10 seconds.

This position also plantar-flexes the ankle and so the anterior tibial muscle will be stretched to some degree.

It may be emphasized by some exercise teachers that to reduce the strain on the metatarso-phalangeal joints (the toes with the bones of the foot) the foot should be held and not the toes.

Stand either free and in balance, or holding on to a partner or wall. Flex one knee and lift the foot of that leg towards the buttock. Grasp that foot with the hand and gently pull the heel of that foot in towards the buttock, at the same time pushing the hip forwards. (This pushing forward of the hip is important in order to achieve a full stretch of rectus femoris which crosses the hip joint.) Keep that thigh pointing downwards, close to and in line with the thigh of the supporting leg. NB. When pushing the hips forwards, keep the lower back straight and do not allow it to curve forwards excessively.

Again, for health-related fitness it would be

Quadriceps Muscles at the Front of the Thigh

Lie face down on the floor. Bend one knee and take hold of the foot of that leg with the hand

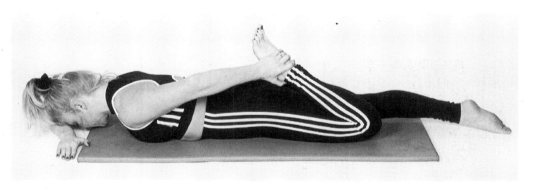

Fig. 135. Prone lying quadriceps stretch.

99

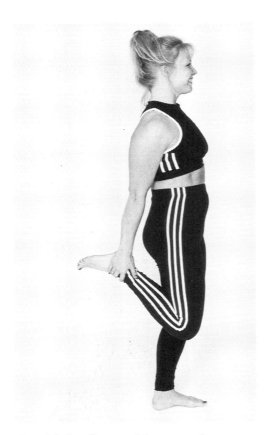

Fig. 136. Standing quadriceps stretch.

tenance of suppleness in this group of muscles, and the consequent flexibility of the knee and hip joints, is essential.

To effect proper relaxation in the hamstrings during stretching, and to ensure maximum safety for the lumbar spine, it is important that correct technique is carried out, and some traditional methods of stretching the hamstrings are no longer recommended.

The hamstring muscles cross both the knee joint and the hip joint, and to stretch the muscles fully the knee must be extended (straight) and the hip flexed (the thigh forwards). However, if a person is particularly inflexible because of tight muscles the full extension of the knee joint in particular may not be possible at first and should not be forced.

Free standing, one foot in front of the other, with the front leg straight and the back leg bent

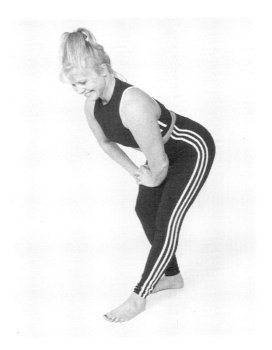

Fig. 137. Hamstrings stretch.

taught that the foot should be held and not the toes. Because of the plantar-flexion of the ankle, the anterior tibial muscles are stretched.

Hamstrings at the Back of the Thigh (biceps femoris, semitendinosus, semimembranosus)

Tight hamstrings can be particularly prone to injury. Therefore the development and main-at the knee, feet facing forwards. Bend forward from the hip joint and support the body weight on the arms by resting the hands on the thigh of the bent leg. The stretch should be felt in the back of the thigh of the front straight leg. Achieve a full stretch by lifting the hips and buttocks backwards and upwards.

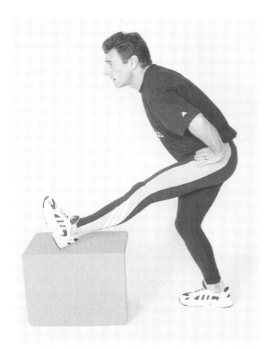

Fig. 138. Hamstrings stretch, one leg supported.

Stand facing a low step, bench, chair or exercise bar (depending on present flexibility and the height required) which will act as a support. Lift one leg and rest it straight on the support. Keep the standing leg slightly 'soft' (knee very slightly bent). Slowly bend forward from the hip joint to achieve a very comfortable stretch and hold the position for about 7 seconds. Then slightly

increase the stretch tension but still within comfort and hold for a further 7 seconds. Increase the stretch tension further, but well within the limits of pain, and hold for a further 7 seconds (the Progressive Stretch Method). The stretch will be felt in the hamstrings of the leg resting on the support. (Do not over-stretch these muscles otherwise contractile tension will develop, the opposite to what we want to achieve.)

With the above hamstring stretching exercise (Fig. 138), if the foot of the supporting leg is turned inwards (which will medially rotate the supporting leg at the hip joint), then the stretch will be emphasized in the outer hamstring muscle (biceps femoris) of the leg being stretched.

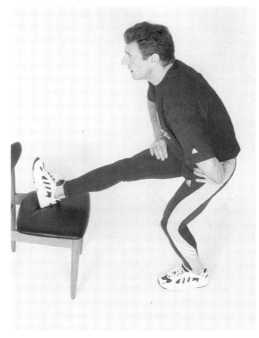

Fig. 139. Hamstrings stretch, one foot turned inwards.

If the foot of the supporting leg is turned outwards (which will laterally rotate the standing leg at the hip joint), then the stretch will be emphasized in the inner hamstring muscles (semitendinosus and semimembranosus) of the leg being stretched.

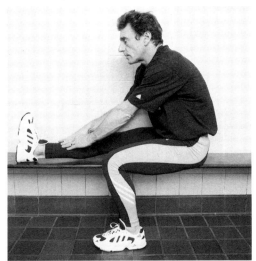

Fig. 141. Hamstrings stretch, seated, one leg outstretched and supported.

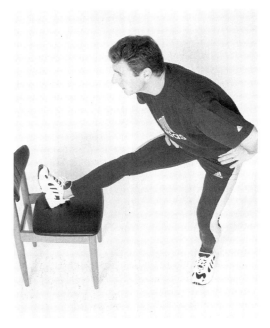

Fig. 140. Hamstrings stretch, one foot turned outwards.

A safe and effective way of stretching the hamstrings is to sit with one leg straight and outstretched along a bench and the other leg bent, down by the side of the bench, with the foot resting on the floor. Bend forwards from the hip joint until a comfortable stretch can be felt in the hamstrings of the straight supported leg and hold for about 7 to 10 seconds for maintenance, or longer using the Progressive Stretch Method for development.

As with the previous hamstring stretches, if

the bent leg by the side of the bench (trailing leg) has the foot turned inwards so that the inside of the thigh rests against the side of the bench, that hip is rotated medially and the stretch will be emphasized in the outer hamstring of the leg resting on the bench.

However, if the foot of the trailing leg is turned outwards, so that the thigh points away from the bench, that hip is rotated laterally, and the stretch is emphasized in the inner hamstrings of the leg resting on the bench.

Another comparatively safe developmental stretch for the hamstrings (although, I feel, having substantial effect on the gluteals) can be achieved by lying supine with the knees flexed and feet resting flat on the floor. Lift one leg and grasp the back of the thigh with the hands. Gently pull that leg towards the chest as far as comfort will allow. Slowly move the hands down the leg and attempt to grasp the leg around the calf region which will enable you to try to extend the knee joint.

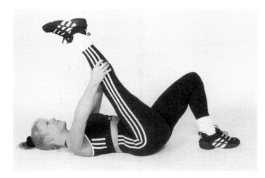

Fig. 142. Supine lying hamstrings stretch.

Many people will find it difficult to extend (straighten) the knee at first and, with a flexed knee, full stretch of the hamstrings is not possible. However, this exercise is safe and effective for beginners concerned with health-related fitness.

The athlete will probably want to use one of the former methods which employ an extended knee and flexed hip.

The traditional method of stretching the hamstrings by standing feet together (or even feet crossed over), legs straight and bending forwards to reach towards the toes, should be absolutely discouraged as ineffective and potentially dangerous for the lower back.

If we were to adopt this position and bounce as well (ballistic stretch), it becomes an extremely dangerous exercise because of the stretch reflex invoked in the hamstring muscles and the consequent possibility of muscle tears. In addition, there would be severe pressure at the pivot point in the lumbar vertebrae, with the possibility of intervertebral disc damage, nerve impingement and back muscle strain.

When we are in a standing position, both the quadriceps at the front of the thigh and

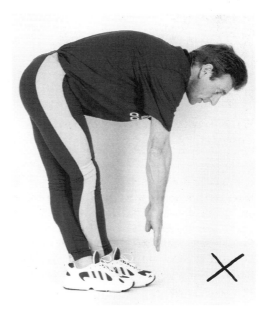

Fig. 143. Traditional standing hamstring stretch (unsafe and not recommended).

Fig. 144. Standing position with feet crossed (unsafe and not recommended).

the hamstrings at the back of the thigh are constantly contracting concentrically (shortening) and eccentrically (lengthening) to hold a standing posture against the force of gravity. Stretch reflex is therefore constantly occurring in both groups of muscles, which results in muscle fibre contraction. If we bend forward the hamstring muscles are stretched, yet still attempt to contract in order to maintain posture. Therefore, we cannot achieve a relaxed lengthening in these muscles, but instead there will be a degree of tension. For that reason it is an ineffective and inefficient method of stretching the hamstrings.

The danger of this position has already been dealt with to some degree in Chapter 10, 'Exercises for the Back'. To bend forwards with straight legs (extended knees) can be very dangerous for the lower back.

Tremendous leverage is applied to the pivot point, which may be the lumbar spine in inflexible people. This results in considerable compression on the anterior (front) aspect of the intervertebral discs, with the possibility of disc prolapse or herniation at the back of the spine. Bulging discs can then impinge on nerve roots which can result in leg pain and back pain.

Also, in this position the extensor muscles of the spine cannot function properly and have little supporting effect and the weight of the upper body is borne by the many tiny ligaments of the vertebral column. Muscles may go into spasm in an attempt to protect the spine, or may even tear in an attempt to contract eccentrically.

Adductor Muscles of the Inner Thigh

It is important to stretch the adductor muscles of the inner thigh as they assist the action of the quadriceps and hip flexors during running, especially when running uphill. The adductor

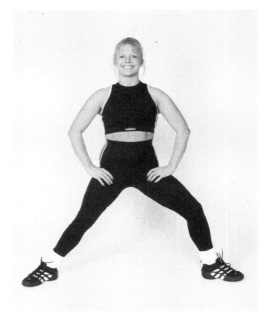

Fig. 145. Adductor muscles stretch, standing.

muscles can be prone to strain and origin inflammation when tight. They are particularly involved in actions such as kicking in football.

The stretch above can be performed by athletes and sports persons, but is often used as part of the pre-stretch and post-stretch components of an exercise to music session.

Stand with the legs fairly wide apart. Turn one foot slightly to the side and bend the knee of that leg so as to lunge to that side. Keep the body facing forwards and do not turn to the lunge side. Keep the other leg straight and the foot of that leg pointing forwards and flat on the floor. Hold for about 7 to 10 seconds. Feel the stretch on the inner thigh of the straight leg. Repeat with the other leg.

Important:
1. Do not lunge too far, which could place excessive stress on the knee joint. Keep the knee

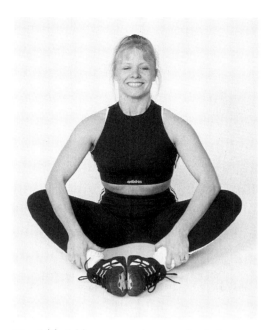

Fig. 146. Adductor muscles stretch, sitting.

Active PNF Stretch of the Adductors

You can also carry out your own PNF stretch in this position: press downwards with the arms for about 7 seconds. Then relax the pressure and try to push the thighs together against the strong resistance of your arms. This produces a strong isometric contraction of the adductor muscles. Hold this contraction for about 4 seconds and then relax for 1–2 seconds. Repeat the stretch, pushing downwards on the thighs and hold for about 7 seconds again. You should experience a greater range of muscle lengthening on the second stretch. This is because the golgi tendon organ in the adductor muscle tendon sensed a very strong contraction and brought about a relaxation in the muscle fibres.

Repeat the procedure a number of times, obtaining greater stretch each time. As it can be fairly tiring to carry out an active PNF stretch, it may be better to recruit the help of a responsible partner as described later on.

Abductor Muscles and the Outer Thigh (gluteus medius, tensor fascia latae and the ilio-tibial band)

The stretching of this region can be very valuable for runners, who may otherwise suffer pain on the outer side of the knee due to inflammation of the ilio-tibial band caused by repetitive friction from tight tissue. Stretching of the abductor muscles can help reduce that tension in the connective tissue.

Sit on the floor with the legs outstretched. Cross the right leg over the left leg with the right foot flat on the floor on the outer side of the left knee. Rest the right hand on the floor behind the body with the arm straight to support the upper body. With the left hand, pull the right knee gently over to the left. Hold for about 7 to 10

of the lunge leg in line with the foot and not beyond the toes.

2. Keep the foot of the straight leg pointing forwards and do not allow it to roll on to the medial (inner) aspect, which could place excessive stress on the big toe joint.

Sit on the floor with the knees bent and the soles of the feet together, back straight. Rest the hands on the inner thighs, just above the knees. Use the arms to press downwards which will further abduct the hip joints and thus stretch the adductor muscles of the inner thigh. (Alternatively, you can take hold of your ankles and use the elbows to force the thighs apart.)

Hold a comfortable stretch for about 20 to 30 seconds, or use the Progressive Stretch Method for development.

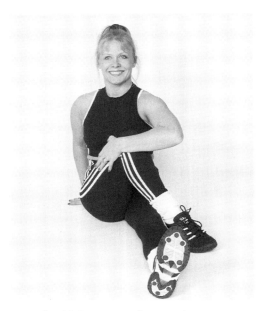

Fig. 147. Abductor muscles stretch.

seconds and feel the stretch in the top of the outer right hip region.

Repeat with the other leg.

Gluteal Muscles of the Buttock (gluteus maximus – hip extensor muscle)

Lie on your back with your knees bent and feet flat on the floor. Keeping one foot on the floor and that knee bent, tuck the other leg up towards your chest and place the hands behind the thigh, linking the fingers. Pull that thigh in towards the chest. Hold that stretch position for about 10 to 20 seconds and feel the stretch in that particular buttock. Repeat with the other leg.

Relax the upper body and keep the head resting back on the floor. Keep the other leg bent with the foot flat on the floor. Do not lift the pelvis too high off the floor.

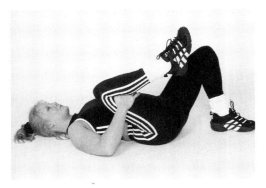

Fig. 148. Gluteal muscles stretch.

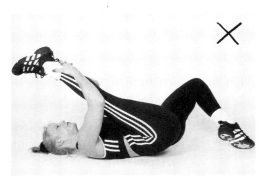

Fig. 149. Gluteal muscle stretch, incorrect method.

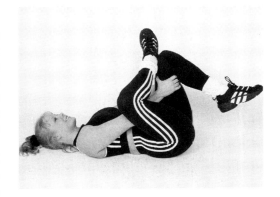

Fig. 150. Alternative gluteal muscle stretch.

Lie on your back with the knees bent and the feet flat on the floor. Lift one leg and cross it over the other leg, which is still resting with the foot on the floor (rest the outside of the ankle of the raised leg on the knee of the lower leg). This will laterally rotate the raised leg slightly. Now lift the lower leg slightly and place the hands round the back of that thigh, linking the fingers. Gently pull that thigh towards the chest and the stretch will occur in the gluteal at the top of the leg which is crossed. Hold for about 10 to 20 seconds. Repeat with the other leg.

Try to relax the upper body and keep the head resting back on the floor.

UPPER BODY

The following stretches are particularly valuable before and after circuit training, exercise to music, resistance training, racket sports, etc.

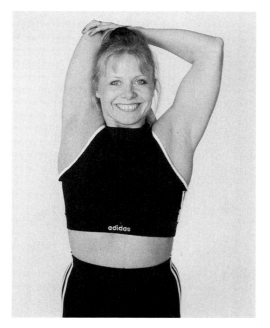

Fig. 151. Triceps standing stretch.

Triceps at the Back of the Upper Arm (and involving latissimus dorsi of the back)

Stand with the knees slightly soft (can also be performed sitting). Lift one arm up and bend the elbow, placing the hand down behind the neck and between the shoulder blades. Lift the other arm and with that hand grasp the original elbow and pull it slightly further backwards. If this is a bit of a strain at first, then that elbow can be pushed with the other hand from the front instead of pulled from above. Hold for about 7 to 10 seconds.

Upper Back (rhomboids)

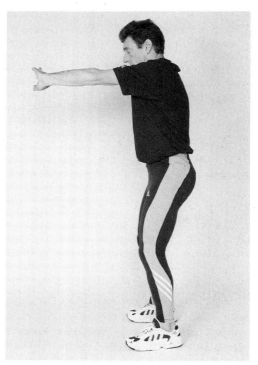

Fig. 152. Upper back (rhomboids) stretch.

107

Stand with the knees slightly soft. Stretch the arms out forwards and link the fingers. Turn the hands palm outwards. Push forwards with the arms and allow the back to curl. Hold for between 7 to 10 seconds and feel the stretch in the upper back.

Chest (pectoralis major)

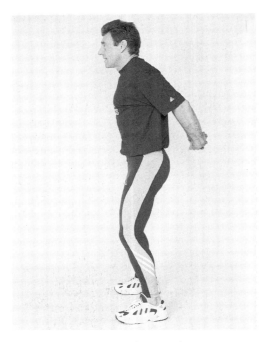

Fig. 153. Chest (pectorals) stretch.

Stand with the knees slightly soft. Place the arms outstretched behind the back and link the fingers. Pull the arms back as far as possible. Hold the position for between 7 to 10 seconds and feel the stretch across the chest and front of the shoulders.

Abdominals

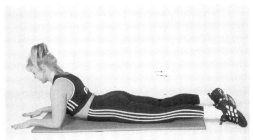

Fig. 154. Abdominals stretch.

Lie prone (face down) on the floor. Place the hands on the floor approximately under the shoulders. Straighten the arms to lift up the upper body, or rest on elbow. Do not push into hyperextension or allow hips to lift from the floor. N.B. It is questionable whether or not this stretch should be performed for health-related fitness as the objective in most cases is to shorten the abdominals. However this stretch influences the anterior ligaments of the spine and reverses anterior disc compression and the effects of repeated forward flexion. It may be effective in remedial cases for certain types of back pain (consult a doctor or physiotherapist).

Waist

Muscles involved include quadratus lumborum (deep), one side of latissimus dorsi, one side of rectus abdominis, and one side of erector spinae.

Stand with the legs apart. Turn one foot slightly outwards and bend the knee of that leg to lunge to that side (do not allow the knee to go beyond the line of the foot). Keep the other leg straight with the foot pointing forwards and flat

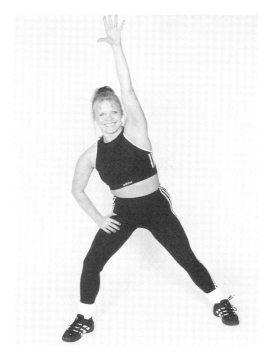

Fig. 155. Waist stretch.

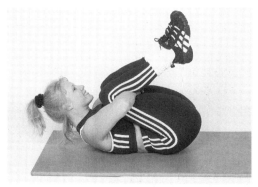

Fig. 156. Back stretch.

abdominals will cause relaxation of the spinal extensors because of a reciprocal inhibition reflex action. Hold for between 7–10 seconds.

Lie on your back with the knees well bent, feet flat on the floor and fairly close to the buttocks. Place the arms outstretched to the sides. Gently lower both knees down to the floor to one side, and then across to the other side. Repeat the movement as many times as desired.

on the floor. Rest the arm on the thigh of the bent, lunge leg to support the body weight. Lift the other arm over the head and lean the upper body towards the lunge side. Hold for between 7–10 seconds. Repeat on the other side.

Mobilizing and Stretching Exercises for the Back

(Muscles involved include erector spinae and obliques; also mobilizes spinal joints).

Lie on your back with the knees tucked towards your chest and hold with the arms. Pull the knees towards the chest as if tucking up. At the same time, contract the abdominal muscles to curl the upper body. The contraction of the

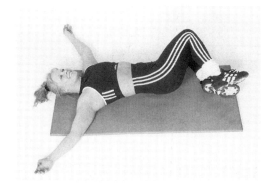

Fig. 157. Spinal mobilizing.

Perform the above exercise carefully and with controlled movements as it is a ballistic stretch.

Lie on your back with the arms outstretched to the sides and the legs straight. Tuck the right

109

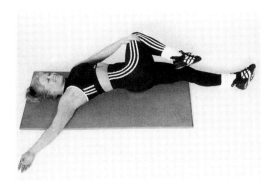

Fig. 158. Abductors and obliques stretch.

leg towards the chest. With the left hand take hold of the outer side of the right thigh close to the knee and pull over towards the floor on the left side of the body. The body will twist and roll over to some degree, but try to keep the right arm and shoulder on the floor.

Psoas Position for the Relief of Lower Back Pain

A lot of the stiffness and pain experienced occasionally in the lower back is because of muscle spasm. The extensor muscles in particular

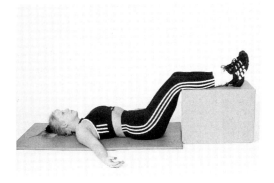

Fig. 159. Psoas position.

protectively tighten up when the spine is put into a potentially dangerous position, as might result from forward bending while load-bearing, adopting an incorrect lifting posture, etc.

To help those tight muscles to relax, the psoas position passively shortens the hip flexor muscles and reduces the tension they normally apply to the lumbar spine.

Lie on the floor on your back with your legs up and over a firm support. If the support is fairly low it will still have an effect, although it is perhaps better if the support is about the height of a chair or bed so that the thighs are almost vertical and at 90 degrees to the trunk. Relax in this position for about 20 minutes, and carry it out two or three times per day for two or three days.

PASSIVE STRETCHES AND PNF STRETCHES WITH A PARTNER

When another person is acting as a partner to help you with passive stretching and PNF stretching, that person must act very carefully and responsibly and must be fully aware of and sympathetic to your limitations.

Moves must be carried out smoothly and slowly, with constant communication between the two persons. Care must be taken not to exert excessive pressure over joints.

Hamstrings (passive)

The subject lies back on the floor with the knees bent and the feet flat on the floor. The partner kneels near the subject's legs, takes hold of one leg which is straightened, and with one hand on the front of the subject's thigh and the other against the back of the subject's heel, raises that leg, flexing the hip. If the partner also allows the heel of the foot of the subject's straight leg to rest

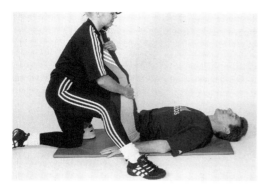

Fig. 160. Passive hamstrings stretch.

on his/her shoulder, then the partner's body weight can be used by leaning forwards and pushing the straight leg up.

Observe the subject's face all the time for any expressions of pain. Do not cause pain to the subject. Coax the subject into relaxing totally. Both subject and partner should continually communicate verbally.

When the subject's limit has been reached, the position is held for 7 to 10 seconds for maintenance, or 20 to 30 seconds for development.

Repeat a number of times, and repeat with the other leg.

PNF Stretching of the Hamstring

Exactly the same procedure is carried out as described above, but this time the stretch position is held for about 7 seconds. Then the subject pushes back with the straight leg as hard as possible against the resistance of the partner for about 4 seconds. This causes a strong isometric contraction in the hamstrings and gluteals which triggers the GTO to relax the muscles. Tension is released for a couple of seconds and then the stretch can be applied again for another 7 seconds.

It should be found that on the second stretch a greater range is achieved.

Passive Stretching of the Adductors

The subject sits on the floor with the legs bent and the soles of the feet together. The subject can either sit free with the arms supporting behind, or could rest his/her back against a wall. The partner kneels in front of the subject, places

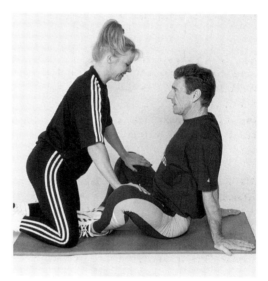

Fig. 161. Passive adductors stretch.

his/her hands on the inside of the subject's knees, and with straight arms allows body weight to press downwards, thus opening the subject's thighs (abducting the hip joints). The position can then be held within the limits of pain for between 7 and 10 seconds for maintenance, or 20 to 30 seconds for development.

Once again, great care must be executed, with empathy and communication between partner and subject.

PNF Stretch of the Adductor Muscles with a Partner

The same procedure is carried out as described above, but this time the stretch is held for about 7 seconds. Then the subject pushes back for about 4 seconds, trying to close the thighs, against the resistance of the partner. The tension is released for a couple of seconds and then the stretch is applied again for another 7 seconds.

It should be found that on the second stretch a greater range is achieved.

13 Dangerous Stretches and Safer Technique

Do's and Dont's

HAMSTRING STRETCHES

Don't attempt to stretch the hamstrings by standing with straight legs and bending forwards reaching towards the toes or the floor. This puts pressure on the lower back, endangers the intervertebral discs and spinal ligaments, and can actually cause the hamstrings to tighten.

Stretch one hamstring at a time, bending the

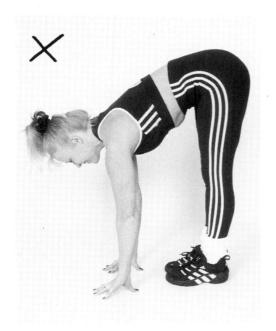

Fig. 162. Hamstrings stretch (unsafe).

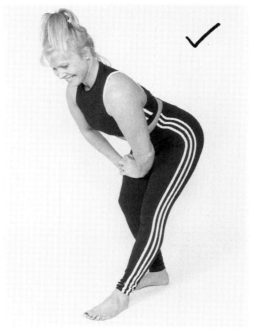

Fig. 163. Hamstrings stretch (safe).

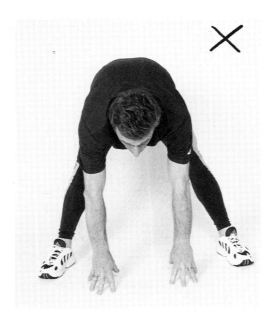

Fig. 164. Hamstrings stretch, legs apart (unsafe).

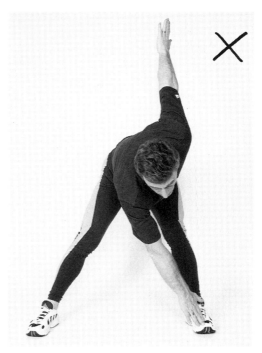

Fig. 166. Hamstrings stretch, legs apart, trunk rotation (unsafe).

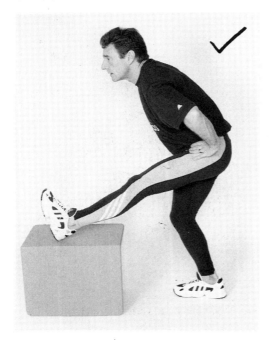

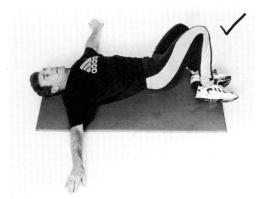

Fig. 167. Spine mobilization, trunk rotation (safe).

Fig. 165 (left). Hamstrings stretch, one leg supported (safe).

other leg and resting the arms on the thigh of the bent leg to support the body weight.

Don't bend forwards with legs apart and straight to touch the floor and bounce, possibly touching in front, between and through the legs. Again, bending forwards with straight legs places pressure on the lower back. The addition of bouncing compounds that pressure and can cause tearing of fibres in the hamstrings or muscles of the lower back.

Use safer methods of stretching the hamstrings such as the one described previously, or lift the leg on to a support and ease into a static stretch.

Don't bend forwards with straight legs wide and rotate the trunk to touch alternate toes. Bending forwards with straight legs places pressure on the lower back and twisting/rotating in

this position produces a sheering force in the intervertebral discs and stress for the spinal ligaments.

Mobilise the spine by performing trunk rotations in a supine lying position and in a controlled manner.

Don't attempt to stretch the hamstrings by adopting a 'hurdle' position. This places stress on the medial aspect of the knee joint and can strain the joint capsule and medial ligament.

Stretch one hamstring at a time in a sitting position but have the other leg bent in a comfortable position. Bend forwards from the hips and not the lower back.

Don't stretch too far when performing a supine-lying hamstring stretch. This tilts and lifts the pelvis which can place stress on the lower back. Also the hamstring muscles may be over-stretched.

Stretch to a comfortable position, keeping the

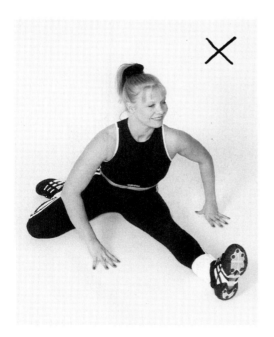

Fig. 168. Hamstrings stretch, hurdle position (unsafe).

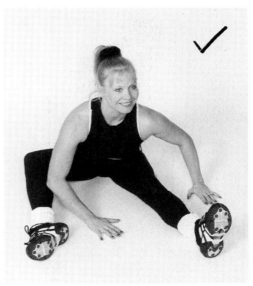

Fig. 169. Hamstrings stretch, sitting, one leg bent (safe).

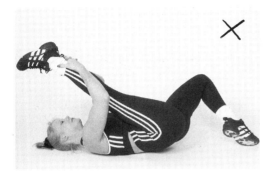

Fig. 170. Hamstrings stretch, too extreme (unsafe).

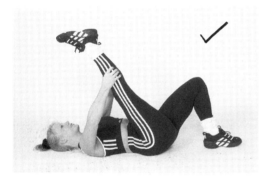

Fig. 171. Hamstring stretch, comfortable (safe).

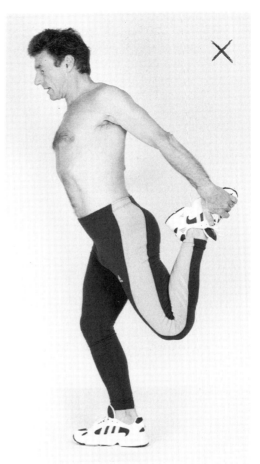

pelvis on the floor. Beginners may wish to hold the back of the thigh. More advanced performers may hold the calf and attempt more extension at the knee.

QUADRICEPS STRETCHES

Don't arch the lower back while pushing the hips forwards during a standing quadriceps stretch.

Press the hips forwards but maintain a straight lower back and an upright posture.

Fig. 172. Quadriceps stretch, standing, back hyperextended (unsafe).

Don't attempt to stretch the quadriceps by kneeling on the feet and then leaning back as far as possible. This hyper-flexes the knee joint under weight-bearing pressure and opens up the knee joint too much, stressing the joint capsule and ligaments.

Stretch the quadriceps in a prone lying position by flexing the knee and holding the foot towards the seat. This eliminates body weight.

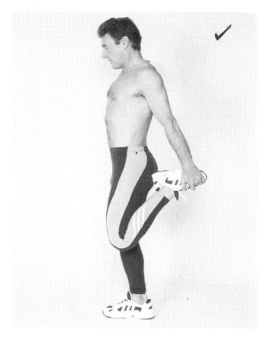

Fig. 173. Quadriceps stretch, standing, upright posture (safe).

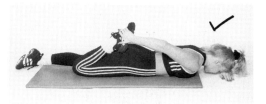

Fig. 175. Quadriceps stretch, prone lying (safe).

CALVES

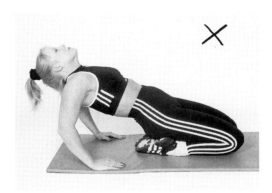

Fig. 174. Quadriceps stretch, kneeling, leaning backwards (unsafe).

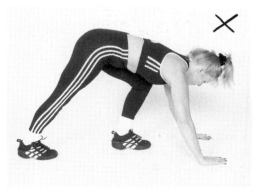

Fig. 176. Calf stretch, sprint position (unsafe).

Don't adopt a 'sprint start' position to stretch the calf. This can be an unstable position for some people, and can increase chest pressure, causing cardiovascular irregularities.

Stretch the calves in either a free-standing position or by pushing against a wall.

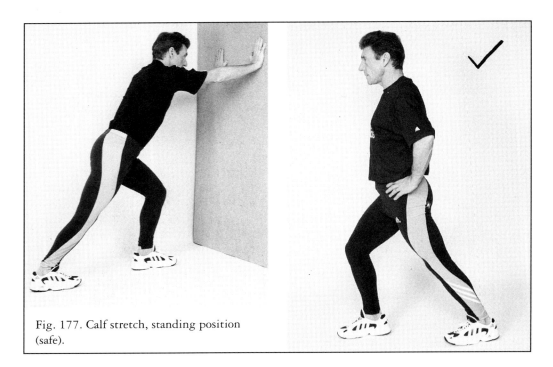

Fig. 177. Calf stretch, standing position (safe).

HIP FLEXORS

Don't lunge too far forwards during a hip flexor stretch so that the front knee becomes hyperflexed.

Lunge so that there is approximately a 90-degree angle at the front knee.

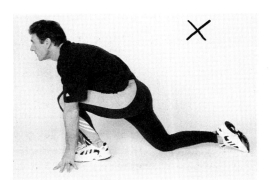

Fig. 178. Hip flexor stretch, lunging far forwards (unsafe).

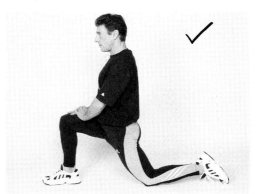

Fig. 179. Hip flexor stretch, lunging at 90 degrees (safe).

ADDUCTORS (INNER THIGH)

Don't lunge too far so that the lunge knee is hyperflexed and the body is leaning forwards.

Lunge so that the lunge knee is flexed to about 90 degrees and the body is kept up straight. Press down slightly on the thigh to emphasize the stretch on that inner thigh.

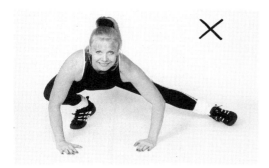

Fig. 180. Adductor stretch, knee hyperflexed, body forwards (unsafe).

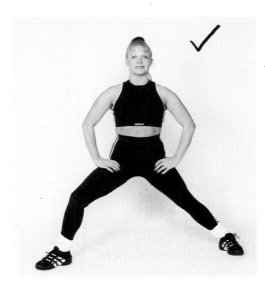

Fig. 181. Adductor stretch, lunge knee at 90 degrees, body straight (safe).

MISCELLANEOUS

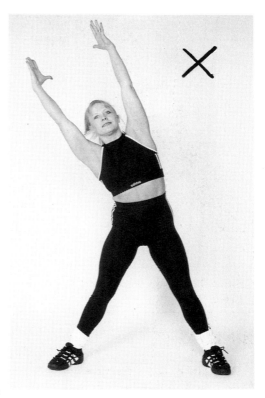

Fig. 182. Side bend, arms above head, quick movement (unsafe).

Don't lean over to the side quickly with arms above the head. This can create a momentum and reduce control, which can result in ligament or muscle strain. The muscles actually try to contract eccentrically because of the stretch reflex.

Lift one arm overhead and support the body weight by resting the other hand on the thigh.

Don't rotate the upper body in a standing position with a bar across the shoulders. This builds up a momentum which can take the spinal joints to their end of range ballistically, tugging

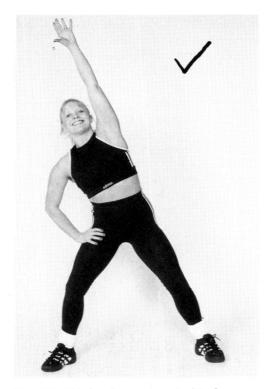

Fig. 183. Side bend, one arm raised (safe).

at the spinal ligaments and creating a sheering force in the intervertebral discs.

Mobilize the spine by rotating the lower body

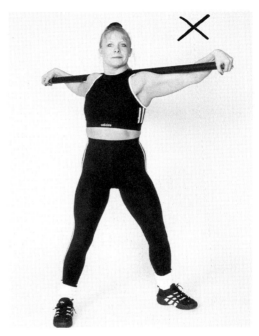

Fig. 184. Upper body rotated, bar across shoulders (unsafe).

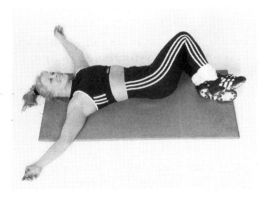

Fig. 185. Spine mobilization, lower body rotated (safe).

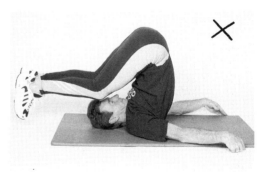

Fig. 186. Plough position (unsafe).

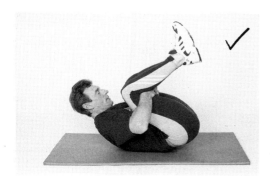

Fig. 187. Spinal muscles stretch (safe).

in a supine lying position. Rotate slowly and in a controlled manner.

Don't attempt the 'plough' position. This places stress on the cervical (neck) vertebrae.

Stretch the muscles of the spine by pulling the knees towards the chest and pulling the head towards the knees. Use of the abdominal muscles causes reciprocal relaxation of the spinal extensor muscles.

Use the stretch below for remedial purposes to reverse anterior disc compression and the effects of forward flexion (if back or leg pain is

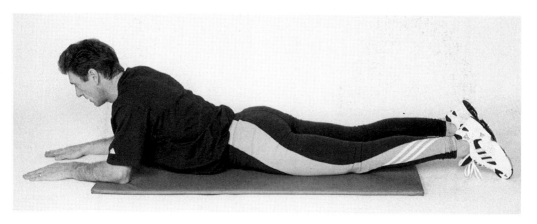

Fig. 188. Spinal extension (safe).

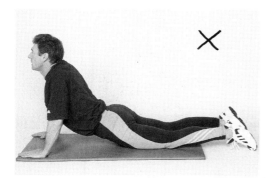

Fig. 189. Hyperextension with hips not supported (unsafe).

present, consult a doctor or physiotherapist). NB. Don't push up into an extreme position.

Don't lower into this position from a press-up position. If the hips are not supported on the floor, compression of the intervertebral discs may result and the possibility of ligament strain.

Don't attempt to mobilize the neck by circling it round. Hyperflexion and hyperextension combined with rotation can compress intervetebral discs and impinge nerve roots.

Bend side to side, forwards/downwards, and rotate to each side separately and in a controlled manner.

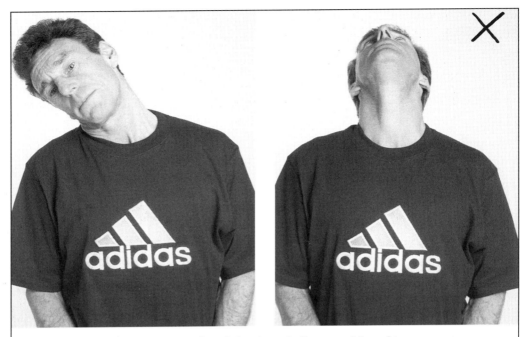

Fig. 190. Neck mobilization, circling round (unsafe).

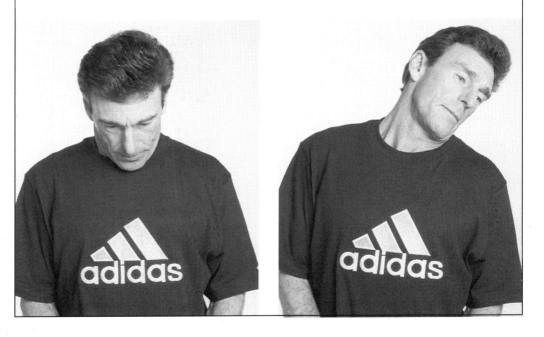

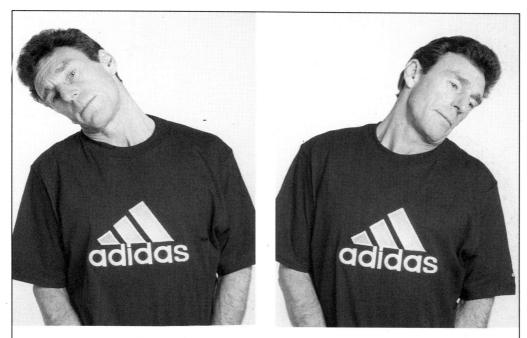

Fig. 191. Neck mobilization, side to side and forwards and downwards (safe).

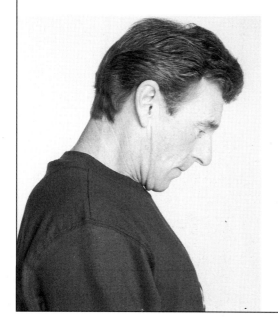

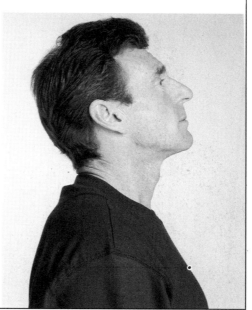

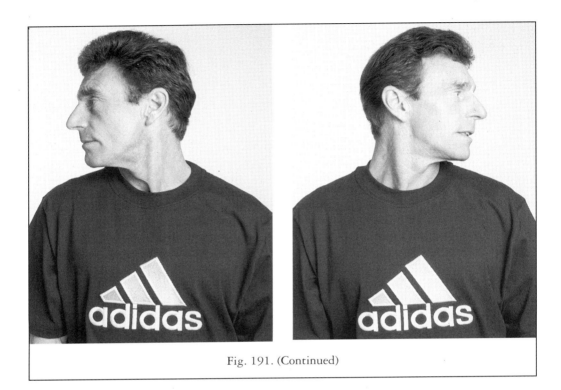

Fig. 191. (Continued)

References

Alter, M.J. (1990). *Sport Stretch*. Leisure Press (Human Kinetics), Champaign, Illinois.

American College of Sports Medicine (ACSM). (1986). *Guidelines for Exercise Testing and Prescription*. Lea and Febiger, Philadelphia.

American College of Sports Medicine (ACSM). (1990). Position Statement on the recommended quantity and quality of exercise for developing and maintaining cardiorespiratory and muscular fitness in healthy adults. *Medicine and Science in Sports and Exercise*. 22 (2).

Anderson, B. (1989). *Stretching*. Pelham Books, London.

Bailey, D. (1996). Legal clinic: coaching and the law. *Sports Industry*. 123 (Jan.), 8–9.

Baird, J. (1996). Posture. *Pro Link*. Feb./March.

Bouchart, C., Shepard, R.J. and Stephens, T. (eds). (1993). *Physical Activity, Fitness and Health: Consensus Statement*. Leisure Press (Human Kinetics), Champaign, Illinois.

Champion, L. (1990a). The key to potentially dangerous exercises. *Pro Link*, June/July, 1–5.

Champion, L. (1990b). Arm movements which cause excessive back extension (hyperextension). *Pro Link*. Aug/Sept.

Chivers, L. (1995). AB training. *Pro Link*, Aug/Sept, 24–25.

Cooper, K.H. (1980). *Aerobics*, Bantam Books, New York.

Cooper, K.H. (1986). *Running Without Fear*, Bantam Books, New York.

Crisp. T. (1997). Exercise addiction: is it a problem? *Pro Link*, June/July.

Cullen, K. (1997a). Exercise watch (abdominals), *Pro Link*, June/July.

Cullen, K. (1997b). Exercise watch (abdominals, part 2), *Pro Link*, Aug./Sept.

Cullum. R. and Mowbray, L. (1989). *Y.M.C.A. Guide to Exercise to Music*. Pelham Books, London.

De Mond, T.E. (1993). Recognising overtraining. *Pro Link*, June/July.

Egger, G., Champion, N. and Hurst, G. (1988). *The Fitness Instructor's Exercise Manual*. David and Charles, London.

Howley, E.T. and Franks, B.D. (1992). *Health and Fitness Instructors' Handbook*. Leisure Press (Human Kinetics), Champaign, Illinois.

Lycholat, T. (1995a). Get back into alignment. *Sports Industry*, 114 (Feb.), 22–23.

Lycholat, T. (1995b). Stretching methods. *Sports Industry*, 115(Mar.) 22–23.

Mitchell, L. (1987). *Simple Relaxation*. John Murray, London.

Mitchell, L. and Dale, B. (1980). *Simple Movement – The Why and How of Exercise*. John Murray, London.

Norris, C.M. (1993). Abdominal muscle training in sport. *British Journal of Sports Medicine*. 27 (1), 19–27.

Norris, C.M. (1994a). Abdominal training; dangers and exercise modification. *Physiotherapy in Sport*. 14 (1): 10–13.

Norris, C.M. (1994b). *Flexibility Principles and Practice*. A. and C. Black, London.

Primos, W.A. (1996). Sport and exercise during acute illness. *The Physician and Sportsmedicine*, 24 (1), 44–52.

Pullig-Schaltz, M. (1994). Easy hamstring stretches. *The Physician and Sportsmedicine.* 22 (2), 115–116.

Rosenbaum, D. and Henning, E.M. (1995). The influence of stretching and warm-up exercises on Achilles tendon reflex activity. *Journal of Sport Sciences*, 13 (6), 481–490.

Smith, B. (1994). *Flexibility for Sport.* Crowood Press, Wiltshire.

Stamford, B. (1995a). How to warm up and cool down your workout. *The Physician and Sportsmedicine*, 23 (9), 97–98.

Stamford, B. (1995b). Safer alterations to outdated exercises. *The Physician and Sportsmedicine.* 23 (6), 87–88.

Index

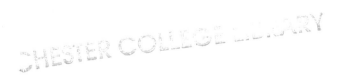